STRESS STRATEGIES

Table of Contents

INTRODUCTION

A Game of Chess

According to the *American Psychological Association's* survey *"Stressed in America"* released in 2015, the top four sources of stress were:

1. *Money*
2. *Work related stress*
3. *Familial stress*
4. *Heath related stress*

The top stressors for 2007, 2008, 2009, and 2010 from the *APA* survey released in 2010 were:

1. *Money*
2. *Work*
3. *Economy*
4. *Family Responsibilities*
5. *Relationships*
6. *Personal Health Concerns*
7. *Housing Costs*
8. *Job Stability*
9. *Health Problems affecting family members*
10. *Personal Safety*

Now, let's think of stress in terms of playing a game of chess. On one side of board we have our opponent: **Stress.**

Labeling the pieces per the *APA* surveys:

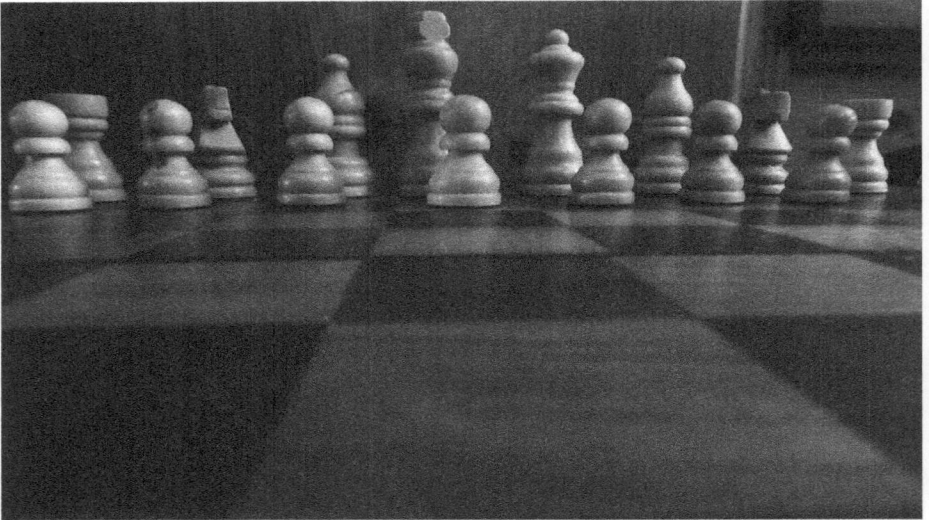

- ❖ **King:** Money
- ❖ **Queen:** Work
- ❖ **Bishop 1:** Familial stress
- ❖ **Bishop 2:** Economic Worry
- ❖ **Knight 1:** Relationships
- ❖ **Knight 2:** Personal Health Concerns
- ❖ **Castle 1:** Housing Costs
- ❖ **Castle 2:** Job Stability
- ❖ **Pawns:** Health Problems affecting family members, personal safety, and other personal stresses

On the other side of the board: **YOU.** More specifically, how you handle stress, what moves you make to react to specific stressors and how well prepared you are to combat these stresses.

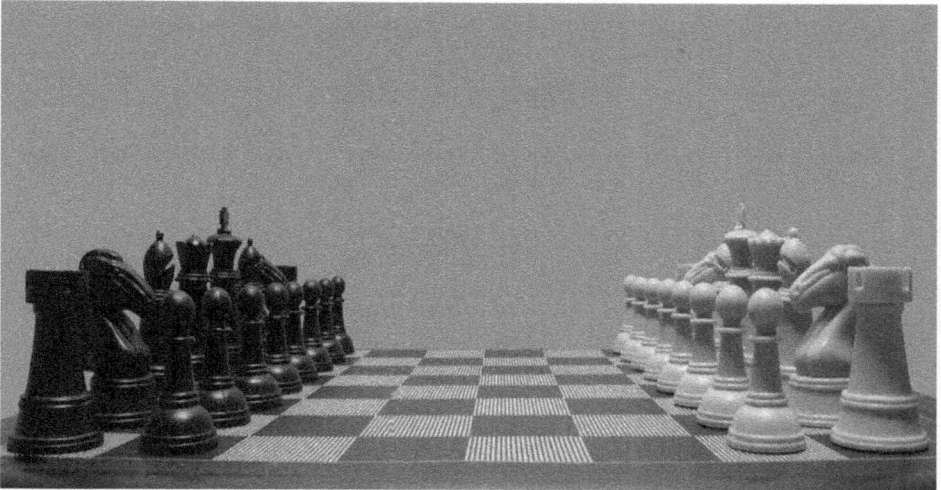

Now that the board is set up, it is time to play chess. When stress makes a move how do you respond to it? If stress moves a pawn two spaces forward, do you move your Queen? Or do you acknowledge that move, while planning your own move with your Bishop? When stress makes a big move with your personal health (Knight 2), what move do you make in response to it?

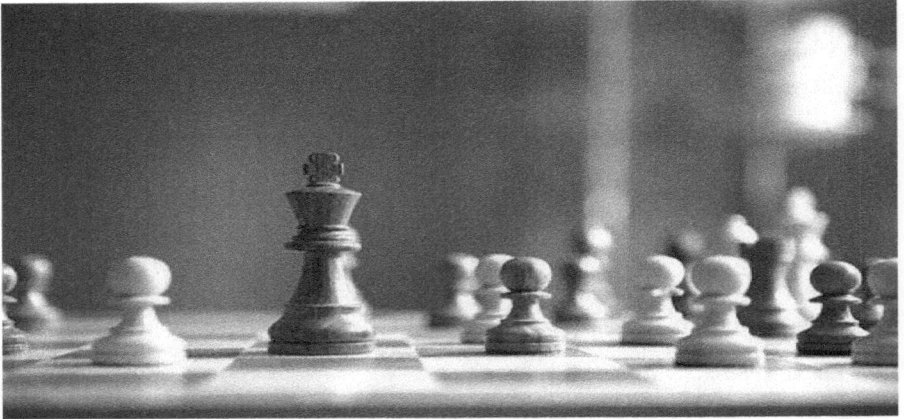

Within this **YOU** vs **STRESS** game of chess, there are smaller games of chess you must play in combatting each individual stress.

For example, you are having an issue with a co-worker. What strategic moves do you make to handle the stress of that situation? You and your spouse are having a spat over their spending habits. What countermoves do you make to overcome the negative behaviors?

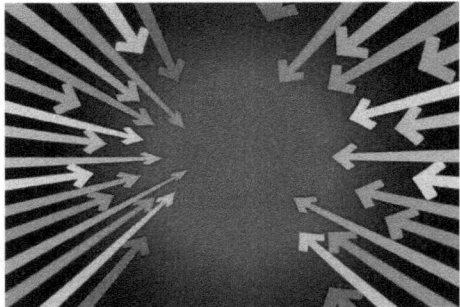

Do you allow yourself to become overwhelmed, paralyzed by the perception that the stress is too great for you to overcome?

According to social psychologist and author Dr. Joseph McGrath, stress is "the interaction between three elements (McGrath 1976):

1. "Perceived demand"
2. "Perceived ability to cope"
3. "The Perception of the importance of being able to cope with the demand"

All three of these elements have one word in common: **perceive.** Just like playing the game of chess, when your opponent, moves their pawn two spaces forward, do you perceive this as a major threat? Do you feel this perceived threat warrants a big countermove? If so, do you have the necessary strategy to counter this?

The 2010 *APA* survey also looked at the physical manifestations of those stressors. These include:

1. Irritability and anger
2. Fatigue
3. Lack of interest, motivation or energy
4. Feeling nervous or anxious
5. Headache
6. Feeling depressed or sad
7. Feeling as though you could cry
8. Upset stomach and indigestion
9. Muscular tension
10. Change in appetite
11. Teeth grinding
12. Change in sex drive
13. Tightness in my chest
14. Feeling faint or dizzy
15. Change in menstrual cycle
16. Erectile dysfunction

If your perception of the demand is too great and your confidence in your ability to cope with the demand is too low, you may be felling like this:

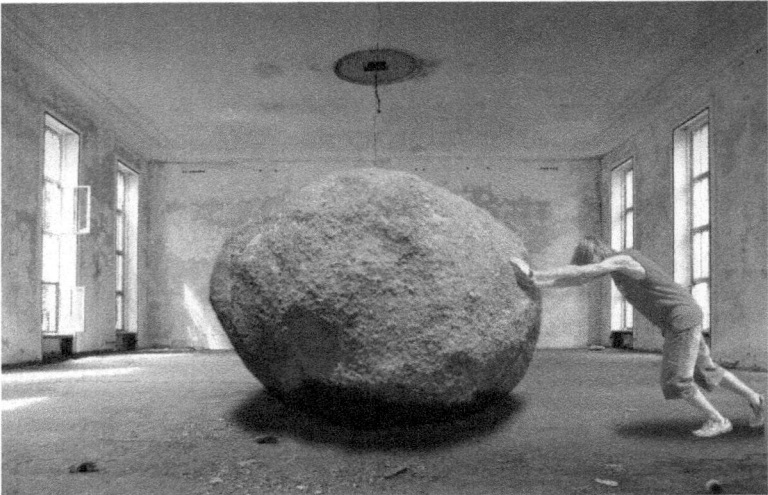

Which may then lead to this:

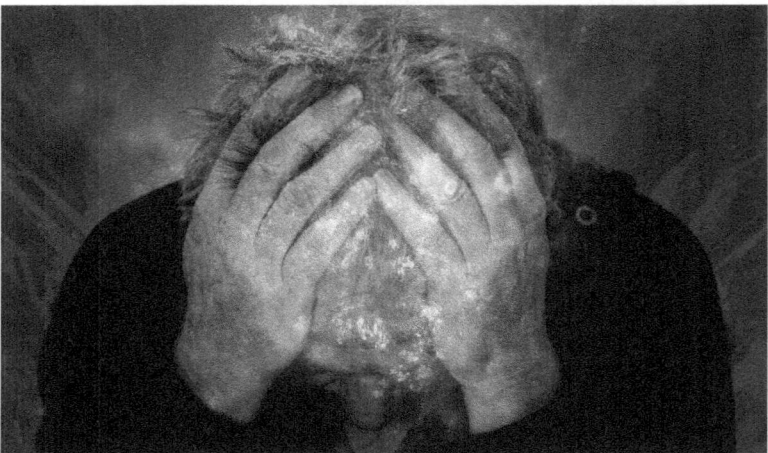

CORTISOL: THE STRESS HORMONE

Normal Cortisol Range Throughout the Day

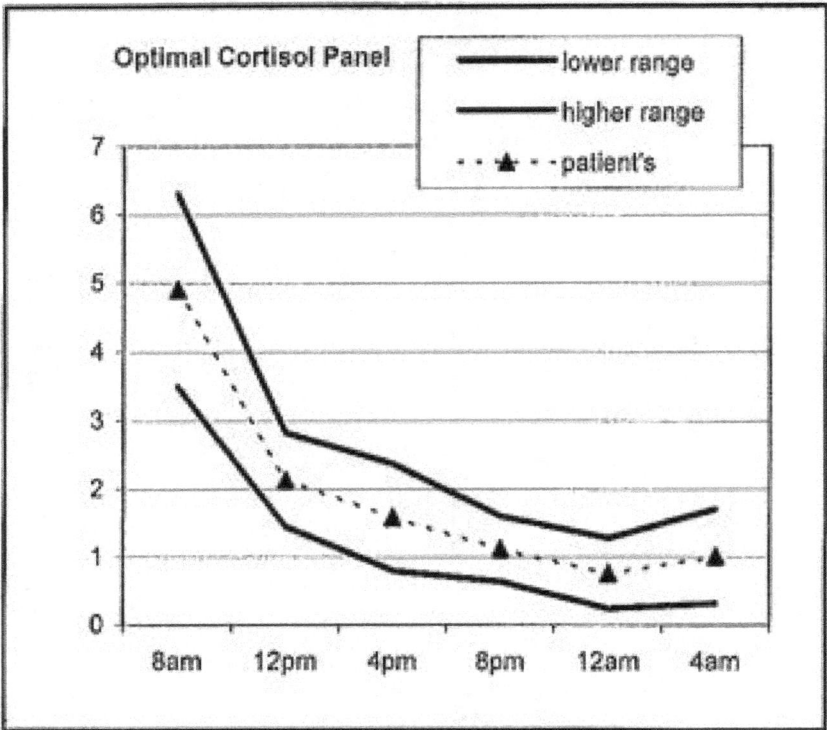

Cortisol is released in diurnal pulsatile patterns throughout the day. There is an average of about 10 secretory bursts per 24 hours.

The major burst occurs just before you wake up, accounting for roughly one half of the daily pulsatile secretion. This is under normal, non-stressful circumstances.

It is a beautiful early spring day and you decide to go for a hike up that mountain you have been eyeing for quite some time. You pack your gear, throw on your hiking boots, strap on your back pack, and head out the door before dawn.

As you begin to ascend the mountain you feel the warm morning sun on your face as it is starting to shine through the trees. You breath in the fresh invigorating forest air. With every breath, you are becoming more energized, feeling more alive.

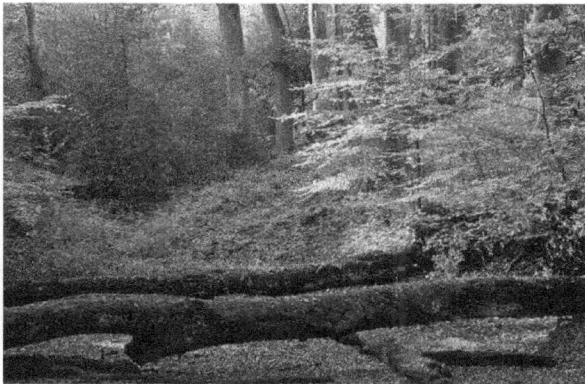

About three hours into your hike a light spring snow begins to sprinkle over the mountain. What a perfect day for a hike.

Up ahead on the snow covered trail you catch a slight glimpse of something moving. Curious, you hike closer toward the movement. Then from out of the woods about fifty feet in front of you...

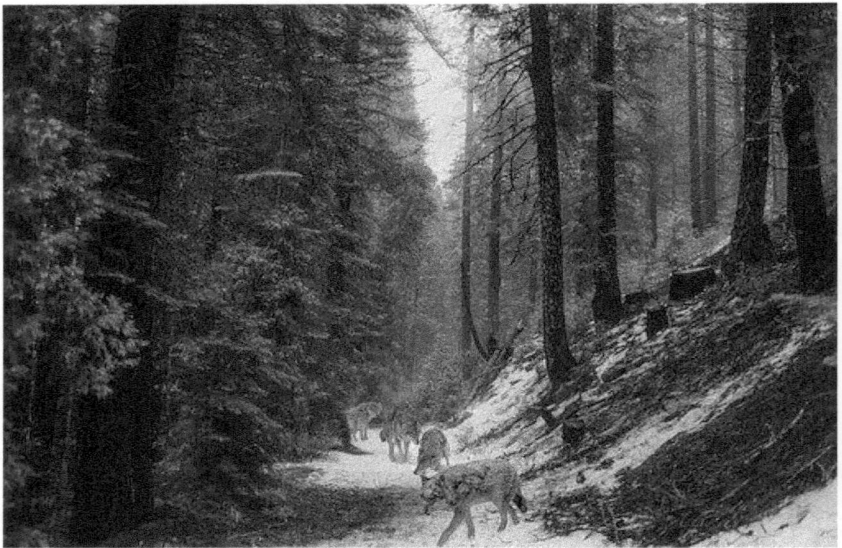

Enter the *Stress Response.*

Stress Response Physiology

Stress Response: The Hypothalamic Pituitary-Adrenal (HPA) System	Stress Response: Sympathomedullary Pathway (SAM) (Fight or Flight)
The **pituitary gland** secretes adrenocorticotropic hormone (ACTH)	The hypothalamus also activates the **adrenal medulla** (Autonomic Nervous System).
ACTH stimulates the **adrenal glands** to produce the hormone **corticosteroid**	The hypothalamus then secretes **ARH** (adrenocorticotrophic releasing hormone)
The **adrenal cortex** releases stress hormones called **cortisol**	Adrenal glands release hormone **adrenaline** (other hormones, including noradrenaline are released into the blood stream as well)
Cortisol is produced is to help bring the body from a state of stress back to homeostasis.	Heart pumps with increased force/rate → raising blood pressure
Vasopressin activates the ducts of the kidneys that are responsible for collecting water to take back some water from the kidneys and minimize the production of urine	Blood vessels in the skin, kidneys, and digestive tract become narrow; increased circulation of free fatty acids; increased output of blood cholesterol
Glucose is released from the liver to be used as energy to combat stressful situation	Increased breathing rate and dilation of airways occurs, so they can supply extra oxygen to the blood and you breathe in and out faster
	Pupils widen to allow for clearer vision; increased brain wave activity
	Adrenaline can cause muscles to tighten, increasing body heat and sweat;

In response to the stress, there is an immune reaction, a hormonal reaction, and a cardiovascular reaction, each affecting the different systems of the body.

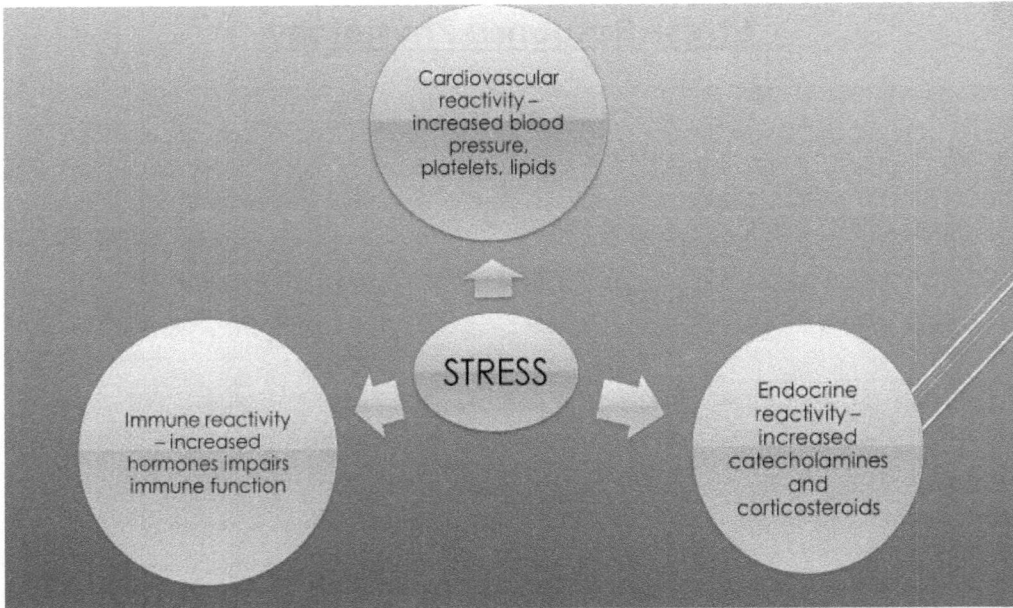

Cardiovascular reactivity – increased blood pressure, platelets, lipids

STRESS

Immune reactivity – increased hormones impairs immune function

Endocrine reactivity – increased catecholamines and corticosteroids

A. **Nervous System:** Fight or flight response, sympathetic nervous system signals body to release cortisol and adrenaline, raising heart rate blood pressure, etc.

B. **Hormonal System:** Adrenal glands release cortisol; Adrenal Medulla releases epinephrine; Liver releases glucose into the bloodstream for fuel

C. **Respiratory System:** Increase in respiration rate as more oxygen needed for working muscles/fight or flight response

D. **Cardiovascular System:** Dilated blood vessels to accommodate for increased heart rate

E. **Musculoskeletal System:** Muscles become tense leading muscle tension, headaches, and strains

F. **Digestive System:** Digestion and excretion are interrupted as well as absorption of nutrients

G. **Reproductive System:** Impacts sexual desire, decreases testosterone, altered menstrual cycle and fertility.

CORTISOL'S EFFECTS ON METABOLISM

increase production of blood sugar so we can have the energy needed to react to the stressful situation. It also helps the blood sugar return to normal when the emergency is over.

Accelerates the breakdown of proteins into amino acids to be used as energy

Shifts cells from CHO metabolism to fat metabolism by increasing lipolysis

Decreases glucose utilization and insulin sensitivity of tissues

Regulates potassium and sodium levels, cortisol returns the acidic/alkaline balance in the body to normal after a stressful situation

CORTISOL'S EFFECTS ON OTHER HORMONES

Cortisol competes with progesterone at progesterone receptor sites creating estrogen dominance

Increased estradiol from estrogen dominance leads to increase in sex hormone binding globulin which decreases free testosterone

Cortisol can shut down the production of TSH and disrupt inactive T4 to active T3 conversion to disrupt metabolism

Can decrease the responsiveness of tissue to thyroid hormone further disrupting metabolism

Can decrease Insulin sensitivity which alters blood sugar regulation leading to excessive glucose in the blood stream.

CORTISOL'S EFFECTS ON IMMUNE FUNCTION

During acute stress higher levels of cortisol result in: Enhanced immunity and enhanced memory. During chronic or prolonged stress the increased level of cortisol result in lower immune response

Cortisol inhibits the release of the mediators of the inflammatory response

Chronically high Cortisol inhibits the production of IL-2 and proliferation of T lymphocytes

Chronic stress Inhibits release of histamine

Studies have shown that people with chronic stress have lower white blood cell counts than people with less chronic stress

CORTISOL'S EFFECTS ON THE BRAIN

The hippocampus is the brain structure primarily responsible for learning and memory. Cortisol decreases and retracts the dentritic growth in the hippocampal area.

Repeated or chronic stress causes dendritic shortening in the medial prefrontal cortex. This results in impairment in attention set shifting

Both acute and chronic stress produce dendritic growth in neurons in the amygdala. The result of include: increased anxiety and increased aggression

Optimism is associated with lower cortisol production and higher heart rate variability

Poor self esteem leads to increased levels of cortisol, inability to regulate cortisol levels under stress – 12-13% loss of hippocampal volume.

Stress causes an increase in ACTH (adrenocorticotropin hormone), leading to more work required of the adrenals to produce more cortisol.

The stress message continues to be sent, causing the adrenal glands to continue the production of cortisol.

*"During the stress response, mind and body can amplify each other's distress signals, **creating a vicious cycle** of tension and anxiety."*

CHAPTER 1: FACTORS THAT AFFECT STRESS/CORTISOL

AGE

"In older adults, notably those reporting high levels of perceived stress, decline in self-esteem has been shown to predict an elevated diurnal cortisol output (34)"

A 2015 study from *Trends in Neurosciences* found that stress was a "frequent psychobiological mechanism" for age related psychosomatic and psychosocial decline (47).

A separate study, this one from the 2013 in *Psychology of Aging*_found that *"stress related psychological and affective dimensions seem to play a role in moderating age-related changes in HPA activity: in a large sample spanning 50 years of adulthood, the increase in cortisol output across the day was shown to correlate with higher levels of average negative affect (46)."*

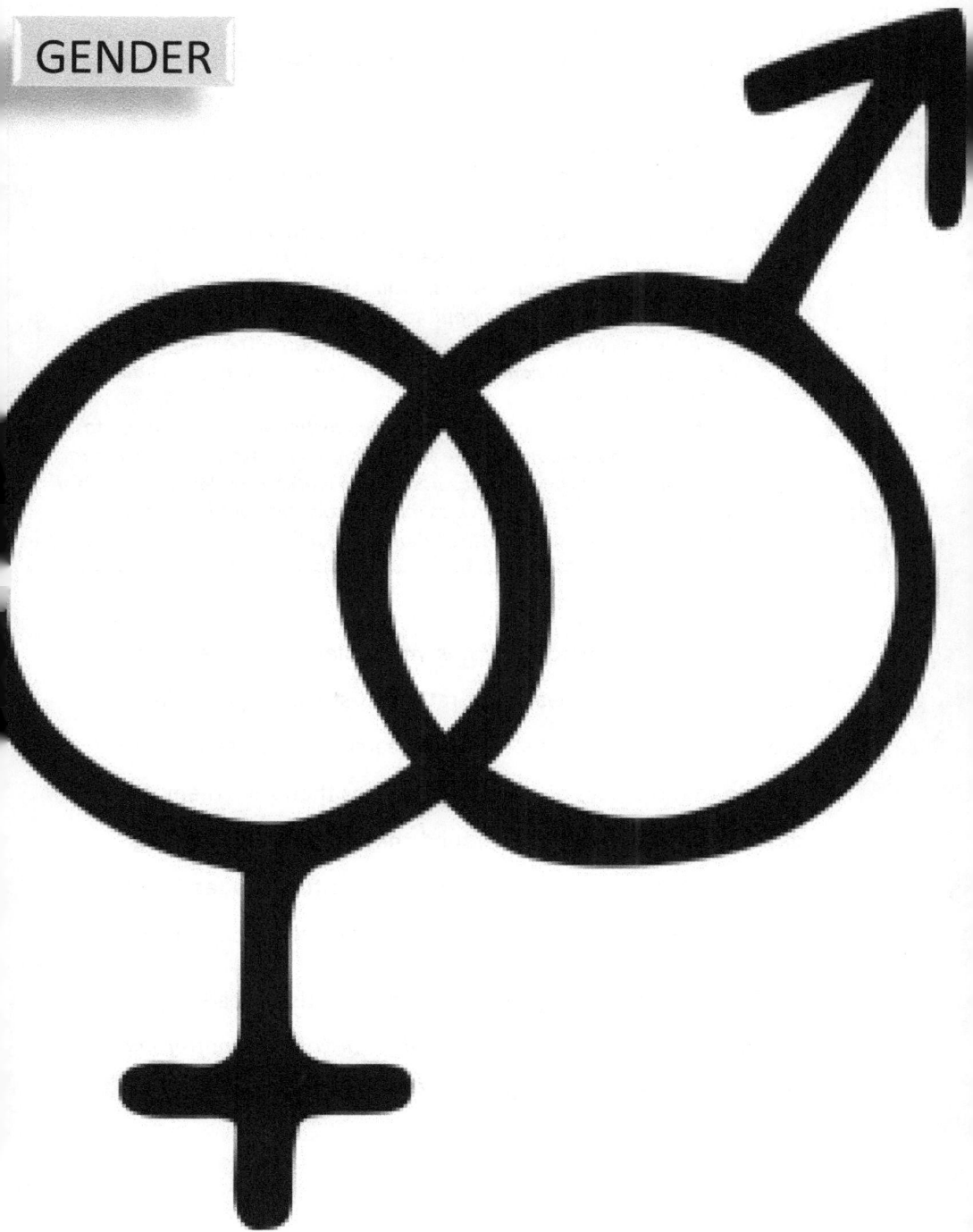

GENDER

Wang J, Korczykowski M, Rao H, Fan Y, Pluta J, Gur R, McEwen B, Detre J. **Gender difference in neural response to psychological stress.** *Soc Cogn Affect Neurosci.* 2(3); Pp 227-239. 2007.

> ➤ *16 male and 16 female subjects*
> ➤ *Had MRI imaging before, during and after mental arithmetic tests under stress.*
> ➤ ***"Men had increased blood flow to right prefrontal cortex and decreased blood flow to the left orbitofrontal cortex while women saw increased blood flow of the limbic system, including the ventral striatum, putamen, insula and the cingulate cortex."***
> ➤ *"The brain activation lasted in both subjects after the tests, but the **response was significantly longer in the female brain. Men had higher cortisol responses."***
> ➤ *"Both men and women's brain activation lasted beyond the stress task, but **the lasting response in the female brain was stronger**. The neural response among the **men was associated with higher levels of cortisol**, whereas women did not have as much association between brain activation to stress and cortisol changes (70)."*

A 2000 study from *Psychosomatic Medicine* looked at the relationship between waist hip ratio and stress response in 59 pre-menopausal subjects. The researchers exposed these women to three days of stressful situations then gave them one day of rest. The researchers found that the women with high waist to hip ratios saw the stressful situations as more threatening/stressful and performed poorly in these challenges.

These women also secreted more cortisol, leading the researchers to conclude that *"central fat distribution patterning is related to greater psychological vulnerability to stress and cortisol reactivity* (15)"

Two separate studies from *Obesity Research* looked at the fat distribution patterning of men and women in response to stress and cortisol. The first, from 1994, had similar findings to the above study. They found that high waist to hip ratio women secreted more cortisol, had poorer coping skills and greater variances in mood reactivity. The researchers observed that cortisol did in fact play a role in the association between stress and abdominal fat distribution (16).

The other study, this one from 1999, found that when compared to women with high and low waist to hip ratios, men secreted more cortisol in response to stress, but had lower mood reactivity and a greater desire to regain control (17).

Finally, a 2006 study from *Psychoneuroendocrinology* may have summed it up best when they observed *that "gender differences in the HPA axis response to stress may partially explain such discrepancies* (27)"

SLEEP LOSS

"Sleep loss could thus affect the resiliency of the stress response and may accelerate the development of metabolic and cognitive consequences of glucocorticoid excess (32)."

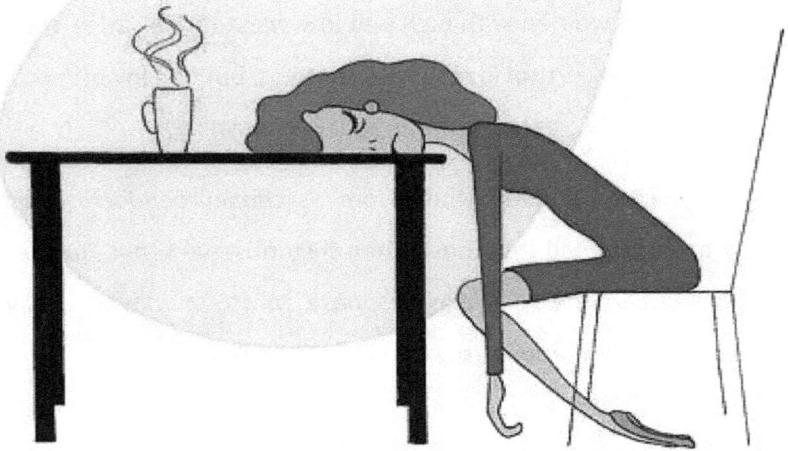

A 1997 study from Sleep evaluated the effects acute total and partial sleep deprivation had on the following days and nights plasma cortisol levels. The researchers found plasma cortisol levels were significantly higher on the second day of total and partial sleep deprivation, when compared to the day after.

Cortisol Levels and Sleep Patterns

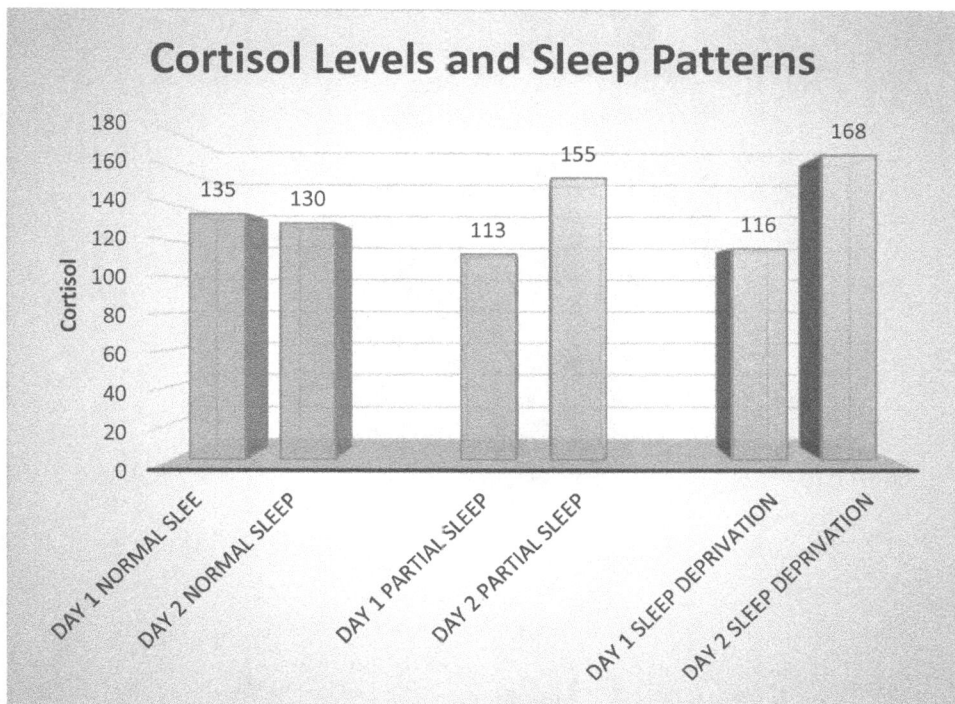

Leproult R, Copinschi G, Buxton O, Van Cauter E. **Sleep loss results in an elevation of cortisol levels the next evening.** *Sleep.* 20(10); Pp 865-870. 1997

OBESITY

"psychosocial stress was associated with greater weight gain among both men and women (Block 2009)"

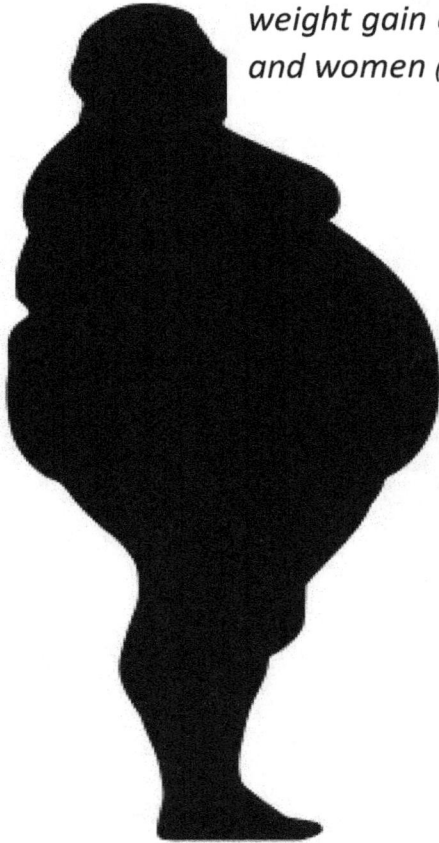

Block J, He Y, Zasiavsky A, Ding L, Ayanian J. **Psychosocial stress and change in weight among US adults.** *The American Journal of Epidemiology.* 170(2); Pp 181-192. 2009.

➢ *Analyzed weight gain of 1355 men and women from 1995-2004*

➢ *"Women had higher levels of baseline psychosocial stress than men in several domains: less skill discretion, less decision authority, more perceived constraints in life, and more strain in relationship with family."*

➢ *"In this nationally representative cohort of US adults followed longitudinally over 9 years,* **psychosocial stress was associated with greater weight gain among both men and women** *with higher baseline body mass indexes if they experienced job related demands, had difficulty paying bills, or had depression or generalized anxiety disorder. Among women with higher baseline body mass indexes,* **perceived** **constraints in life and strain in relations with family also were associated with greater weight gain.** *Among men with higher baseline body mass indexes, lack of skill discretion or decision authority at work was associated with greater weight gain."*

➢ **"Normal weight women with major depression had more than twice the cortisol level and intraabdominal fat as those without depression."**

FOOD/DIET

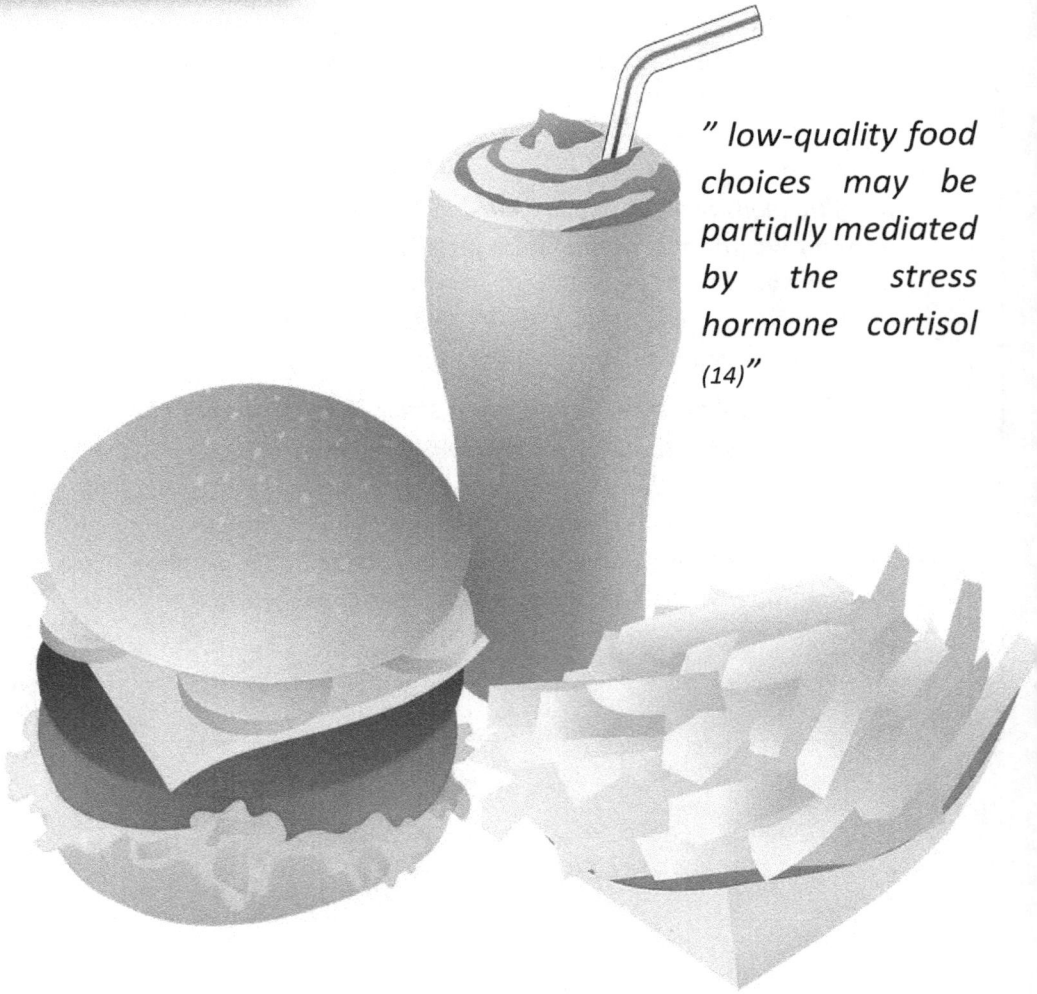

" low-quality food choices may be partially mediated by the stress hormone cortisol (14)"

Counting calories is stressful. In a 2010 study, researchers separated female subjects into four separate groups:

- ➢ **Group 1:** 1200kcal/day dieting group that counted calories
- ➢ **Group 2:** 1200kcal/day dieting group with no counting
- ➢ **Group 3:** No diet but calorie monitoring/counting
- ➢ **Group 4**: Control

The researchers found that both calorie restriction groups had increased cortisol, as the dieting was seen to be a stress on the body. The group that counted calories had higher cortisol and levels of perceived stress than the group that did not.

A 2000 study from *Physiology and Behavior* found that during stressful situations, those subjects with high stress levels responded to high carb meals with a lower cortisol and greater serotonin. The researchers concluded that as an adaptation to these greater stress levels, the subjects had an altered serotonin response to carb rich foods in high stress situations.

In 2010 researchers studied the effects different macronutrients had on cortisol levels in ten healthy male subjects. Over a four-day period, the men had a different macronutrient rich shake for lunch, while having their cortisol levels measured for three hours prior and after ingestion. The researchers found that the protein and fat dense lunches caused

When 27 type one diabetics and 27 non-diabetic healthy control subjects had their cortisol, levels measured against their three-day dietary food journal researchers found that "poor blood sugar management and low quality food choices may be partially mediated by the stress hormone cortisol (14)."

Per a 2015 study, the frequency and circadian timing of eating can cause an increase in both cortisol and inflammatory biomarkers. In other words, eating at the wrong times can negatively impact cortisol levels (39).

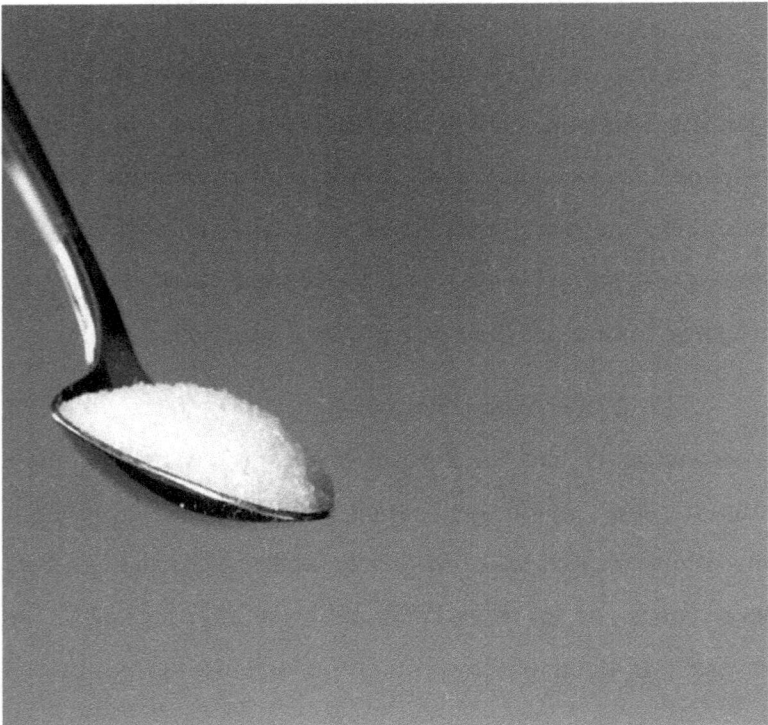

Did you know that the average daily consumption of high fructose corn syrup in the U.S. is about 50 grams per person? Did you also know that mercury was found in nearly 50% of the samples of high fructose corn syrup taken in a 2009 study? The study, from Environmental Health collected high fructose corn syrup samples from three different manufacturers found nine of the twenty samples to contain 0.005 to 0.570 micrograms of mercury per gram of high fructose corn syrup (13).

Per the January 2009 *Institute for Agriculture and Trade Policy* report, mercury was detected in one third of fifty-five popular brand name foods and beverages that have high fructose corn syrup listed as the first or second ingredient on the label. Included in this list of products was Quaker, Hershey's, Kraft and Smuckers.

High Fructose Corn Syrup

- Most is manufactured from genetically modified corn
- Higher in fructose and sweeter than table sugar
- Fructose causes a slower rise in insulin and blood sugar than glucose or sucrose. The problem with this is it leads to dysregulation in leptin levels, which then alters the satiety signal to the brain. This potentially causes us to eat more and because we are still hungry (67)."

According to a 2010 study when the same number of calories were consumed, subjects ingesting high fructose corn syrup had significantly greater weight gain, serum triglycerides, and body fat accumulation about the abdominal region (3).

A group of subjects ingesting 25% of their calories in high fructose corn syrup saw up to a 15% increase in LDL after only two weeks (61) When a group of subjects ingested 25% of their calories as fructose or glucose for ten weeks, the researchers found the subjects consuming fructose had higher serum triglycerides, higher LDL, higher overall cholesterol, and more body fat accumulation (60). A separate study from 2011 had similar findings (62).

Per a 2012 study from *Metabolism*, when subjects consumed 24 oz. of high fructose corn syrup or sucrose drink, the researchers found both a rise in systolic blood pressure and uric acid levels (30).

High fructose corn syrup has also been linked to cancer. Per a 2010 study in *Cancer Research*, *"cancer cells can readily metabolize fructose to increase proliferation. They have major significance for cancer patients given dietary refined fructose consumption, and indicate that efforts to reduce refined fructose intake or inhibit fructose-mediated actions may disrupt cancer growth (33)"*

Food Allergies

A 2011 study from The Journal of Allergy and Clinical Immunology observed that *"salivary cortisol level in the evening was associated with food allergy."* The study stated further that there is "a role of an altered hypothalamic-pituitary-adrenal axis in the etiological process of allergies (64)."

Soy Protein

A 2013 study from the *Journal of the American College of Nutrition* looked at the testosterone, cortisol, and estradiol concentrations in men drinking either soy or whey protein drinks. After fourteen days, the researchers found higher cortisol and lower testosterone in the men drinking soy protein.

THE ROLE OF CORTISOL IN FOOD ALLERGIES

Cortisol, secreted by the adrenal glands, plays a key role in modulating body's inflammatory reaction.

Histamine (and other pro-inflammatory biomarkers) is released in response to food allergies

Histamine is therefore mediated by cortisol.

More allergic reaction to foods, more pro-inflammatory histamine release, more cortisol produced by adrenal glands to combat the inflammation.

As this becomes chronic, there may be less tissue sensitivity to the cortisol or the adrenal glands may become overworked and produce less cortisol, leading to greater and greater reactions to foods.

GRASS FED VS GRAIN FED MEAT

- McAfee A, Mcsorley E, Cuskelly G, Fearon A, et al. **Red meat from animals offered a grass fed diet increases plasma and platelet n-3 PUFA in healthy consumers.** *The British Journal of Nutrition.* 105(1); Pp 80-89. 2011.

    - Green/grass fed meat has been found to have higher concentrations of N-3 LC-PUFA (long chain polyunsaturated omega 3 fatty acids)

- Daley C, Abbott A, Doyle P, Nader G, Larson S. **A review of fatty acid profiles and antioxidant content in grass fed and grain fed beef.** *Nutrition Journal.* 9(10); Pp 1-12. 2010.

    - Grass fed meat had higher levels of antioxidant CLA (conjugated linoleic acid) and less palmitic and myristic acid.

- Ponnampalam E, Mann N, Sinclair A. **Effect of feeding systems on omega-3 fatty acids, conjugated linoleic acid and trans fatty acids in Australian beef cuts; potential impact on human health.** *Asia Pacific Journal of Clinical Nutrition.* 15(1); Pp 21-29. 2006.

    - Grain fed animals have been found to have much greater levels of pro-inflammatory omega-6 fatty acids and trans fats.

ALCOHOL

An increased number of alcohol units consumed per week and heavy drinking are associated with increased cortisol levels (2).

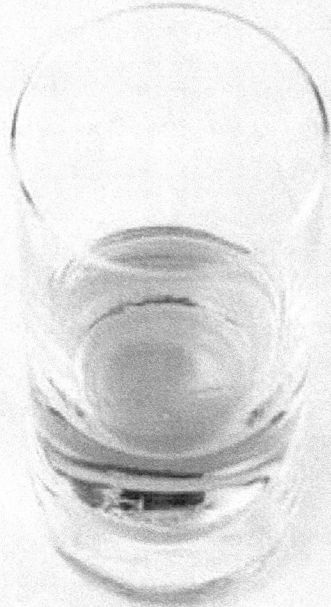

A 2008 study on the relationship between alcohol consumption and cortisol secretion, the researchers observed that "alcohol consumption had a positive relationship with cortisol release over the day (2)."

The researchers also found differences between men and women, with the strongest predictor of cortisol in men being the amount of alcohol consumed per week, whereas women's cortisol was affected by all three alcohol consumption measures used in the study.

Effect	Scientific Literature
Acute alcohol intoxication (roughly 5 drinks in one hour for 160lb man) increases blood cortisol levels	Spencer R, Hutchinson K. **Alcohol, aging, and the stress response.** *Alcohol Research and Health*.23(4); Pp 272-283. 1999.
Chronic alcohol intoxication raises blood cortisol levels	Spencer R, Hutchinson K. **Alcohol, aging, and the stress response.** *Alcohol Research and Health*.23(4); Pp 272-283. 1999.
Withdrawal from alcohol causes alterations in cortisol leading to symptoms often seen in alcohol withdrawal	**Alcohol, the brain, and behavior.** *Alcohol Research and Health.* 24(1); Pp 12-16. 2000.
Alcohol increased cortisol, blood pressure and noradrenaline levels	Ireland M, Bandongen R, Davidson L, Beilin L, Rouse I. **Acute effects of moderate alcohol consumption on blood pressure and plasma catecholamines.** *Clin Sci (Lond).* 66(6); Pp 643-648. 1984.
Alcohol withdrawal can decrease testosterone	Ylikahri R, Huttunen M, Harkonen M. **Hormonal changes during alcohol intoxication and withdrawal.** *Pharmacol Biochem Behav.* 13(1); Pp 131-137. 1980.
Acute and chronic alcohol intoxication have been linked to decreased growth hormone levels	Emanueale N, Emanuell M. **The Endocrine System: Alcohol alters critical hormonal balance.** *Alcohol, Health, and Research World.* 21(1); Pp 53-64. 1997.
Stress, anxiety, depression, mood disturbances, seizures, delirium and indecisiveness from alcohol withdrawal	Trevisan L, Boutros N, Petrakis I, Krystal J. **Complications of alcohol withdrawal.** *Alcohol Research and Health.* 22(1); Pp 61-66.1998
As Serotonin influences the award response from alcohol, acute alcohol consumption spikes the release of serotonin in the brain	Lovinger D. **Serotonin's role in alcohol's effects on the brain.** *Alcohol Health and Research World.* 21(2); Pp 114-120. 1997.
Serotonin levels may be decreased for up to two weeks following alcohol intoxication	Lovinger D. **Serotonin's role in alcohol's effects on the brain.** *Alcohol Health and Research World.* 21(2); Pp 114-120. 1997.
Dopamine a neurotransmitter responsible for alcohol cravings, and its release is spiked with alcohol ingestion.	Chiara G. **Alcohol and dopamine.** *Alcohol, Health, and Research World.* 21(2); Pp 108-113. 1997.

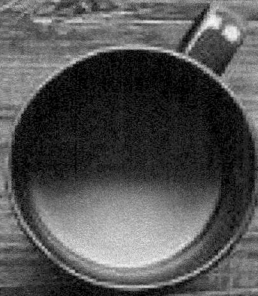

CAFFEINE

Cortisol levels spiked roughly 30% within one hour of consumed the equivalent of 2-3 cups of 2-3 cups of coffee (35)"

A 2005 study from *Psychosomatic Medicine* had subjects consume either 0, 300 mg, or 600 mg of caffeine for four weeks. The researchers found that consuming caffeine multiple times a day led to significantly higher afternoon cortisol levels (36).

DEHYDRATION

"Cortisol levels were greater when dehydrated regardless of the exercise intensity (38)"

A study from the 2006 *International Journal of Sports Medicine* looked at the effects running intensity and dehydration had on testosterone, cortisol, and the testosterone: cortisol ratio. The researchers had 9 male runners perform 4 different 10-minute treadmill protocols: hydrated at 70% intensity, dehydrated at 70%, hydrated at 85% intensity, and dehydrated at 85%. They found cortisol levels were highest in the dehydrated protocols regardless of intensity (38). A 2015 study from *The American Journal of the Medical Sciences*, this one on elite level wrestlers had similar findings (25).

OMEGA-3 DEFICIENCY

"studies reported that the response to chronic stress can be modulated by the omega-3 fatty acid supply (21)"

A 2003 study from Diabetes and Metabolism looked at the effects roughly 7 grams of fish oil/day for three weeks would have on stressful situation induced cortisol and catecholamine levels. The researchers found that the fish oil significantly mediated cortisol while lowering perceived stress levels (10).

A more recent study from 2014 observed that *"EPA may regulate the HPA axis dysfunction associated with depression by reducing corticotrophin releasing factor expression and corticosterone secretion (21)."*

HOUSEHOLD CHEMICALS

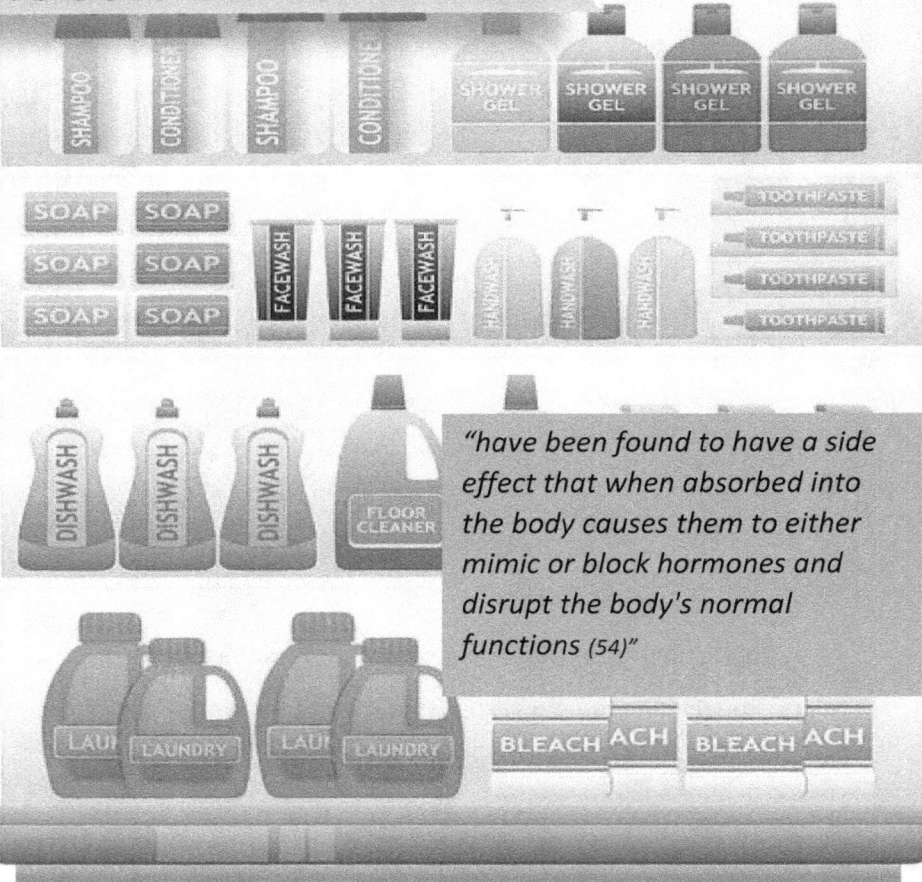

SHAMPOO · CONDITIONER · SHAMPOO · CONDITIONER · SHOWER GEL · SHOWER GEL · SHOWER GEL · SHOWER GEL

SOAP SOAP · SOAP SOAP · SOAP SOAP · FACEWASH · FACEWASH · FACEWASH · HANDWASH · HANDWASH · HANDWASH · TOOTHPASTE · TOOTHPASTE · TOOTHPASTE · TOOTHPASTE

DISHWASH · DISHWASH · DISHWASH · FLOOR CLEANER

"have been found to have a side effect that when absorbed into the body causes them to either mimic or block hormones and disrupt the body's normal functions (54)"

LAU LAUNDRY · LAU LAUNDRY · BLEACH ACH · BLEACH ACH

Per a 2009 study from Endocrine Review *"endocrine disruptors have effects on male and female reproduction, breast development and cancer, prostate cancer, neuroendocrinology, thyroid, metabolism and obesity, and cardiovascular endocrinology. Results from animal models, human clinical observations, and epidemiological studies converge to implicate EDCs as a significant concern to public health (11)".*

The study further states *"EDCs represent a broad class of molecules such as organochlorinated pesticides and industrial chemicals, plastics and plasticizers, fuels, and many other chemicals that are present in the environment or are in widespread use (11)."*

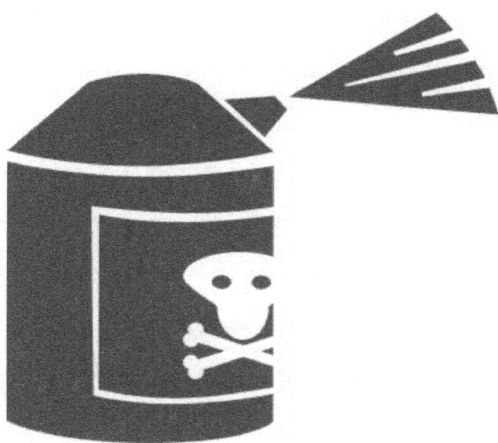

A separate study, this one from 2011 looked at the susceptibility to certain diseases with exposure to these endocrine disrupting chemicals. The authors express that endocrine disruptors *"have been found to have a side effect that when absorbed into the body causes them to either mimic or block hormones and disrupt the body's normal functions. This disruption can occur by altering normal hormone levels, inhibiting or stimulating the production of hormones, or changing the way hormones travel through the body, thus affecting the functions that these hormones control (54)."*

The authors state further *"less well known mechanisms of action of EDCs include direct effects on genes_and their epigenetic impact (54)."*

On a side note, a third study, a 2001 study from the International Journal of Cancer looked at the effects sunscreen had on skin cancer protection and the development of malignant melanoma. They found that *"persons who used sunscreens did not have a decreased risk of malignant melanoma. Instead, a significantly elevated odds ratio (OR) for developing malignant melanoma after regular sunscreen use was found, adjusted for history of sunburns, hair color, frequency of sunbathing during the summer, and duration of each sunbathing occasion (71)."*

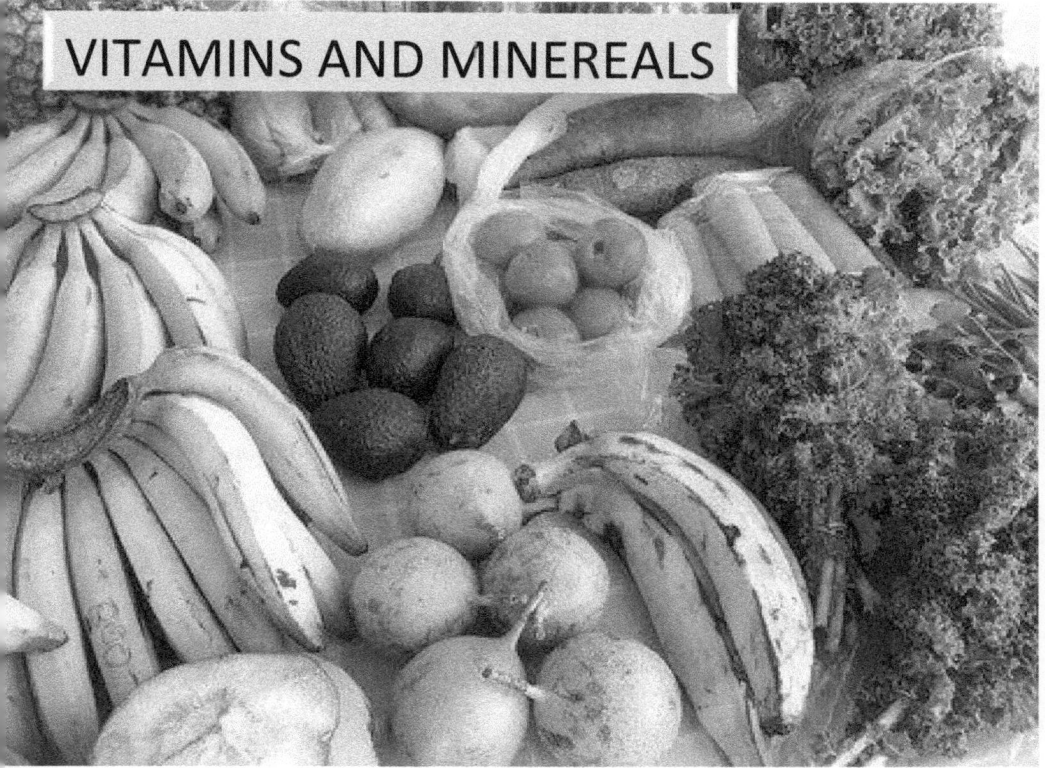

VITAMINS AND MINEREALS

According to a 2013 study from *Nutrients* in which subjects were given a multivitamin or placebo for sixteen weeks, *"supplementation was found to be associated with changes in the cortisol awakening response after 16 weeks (5)."* The researchers found a strong correlation between the cortisol awaking response and folate and B6.

Magnesium has been a widely-studied mineral with regards to its effects on cortisol and the stress response. A 2012 study from *Neuropharmacology* expressed *"reduced magnesium levels are associated with different facets of anxiety behavior. Hence, an inverse relationship between magnesium and anxiety is suggested by these data (53)."*

The same study goes on to state further *"this study proves that in an animal model magnesium deficiency induces anxiety and dysregulation of the way the hypothalamus-pituitary-adrenal axis works." "The HPA axis is often impaired in depression and anxiety as well as chronic fatigue syndrome creating too much cortisol as a manifestation of stress. It's not specifically known what comes first, stress or HPA dysregulation. This is a very important animal model proving the serious effects of magnesium deficiency as the possible cause of HPA axis dysregulation (53)."*

A 2010 study found that by simply adding magnesium to the diets of poor sleepers, their stress levels went down while their quality of sleep went up (45).

Per a study from 2010 in *Magnesium Research* found magnesium to play an important role in the regulation of both cortisol and inflammation (49).

A 1995 study from the *European Journal of Endocrinology* found that Thyroid hormone and cortisol elevate and drop in tandem (58). It is important to point out that deficiencies in certain minerals plays a significant role in thyroid dysfunction. For example, a study from *The Journal of Clinical Endocrinology and Metabolism* found that low Ferritin (stored form of iron) was a cause of thyroid dysfunction (26). Iron is also a building block of the enzyme that is responsible for the initiation of the synthesis of thyroid hormone (58).

Vitamin D deficiency has also been linked to stress response and cortisol. Per a 2012 study by Quraishi and Camargo *"Variations in individual patient responses to acute stress and critical illness may therefore depend on the degree of vitamin D insufficiency and extent of tissue requirement (48)."*

The VDR, or vitamin D receptor, may be affected by cortisol levels. A study from the 2011 *Best Practices and Research Clinical Endocrinology and Metabolism* expressed that a deficiency in vitamin D may exist in acute stress as well as critical illnesses (31). If the tissue receptors are not up-taking the vitamin D, then it will potentially remain in an inactive form in the body.

Quick Tip:

Magnesium has been found to play a role in converting vitamin D from its inactive form to its active form (19)

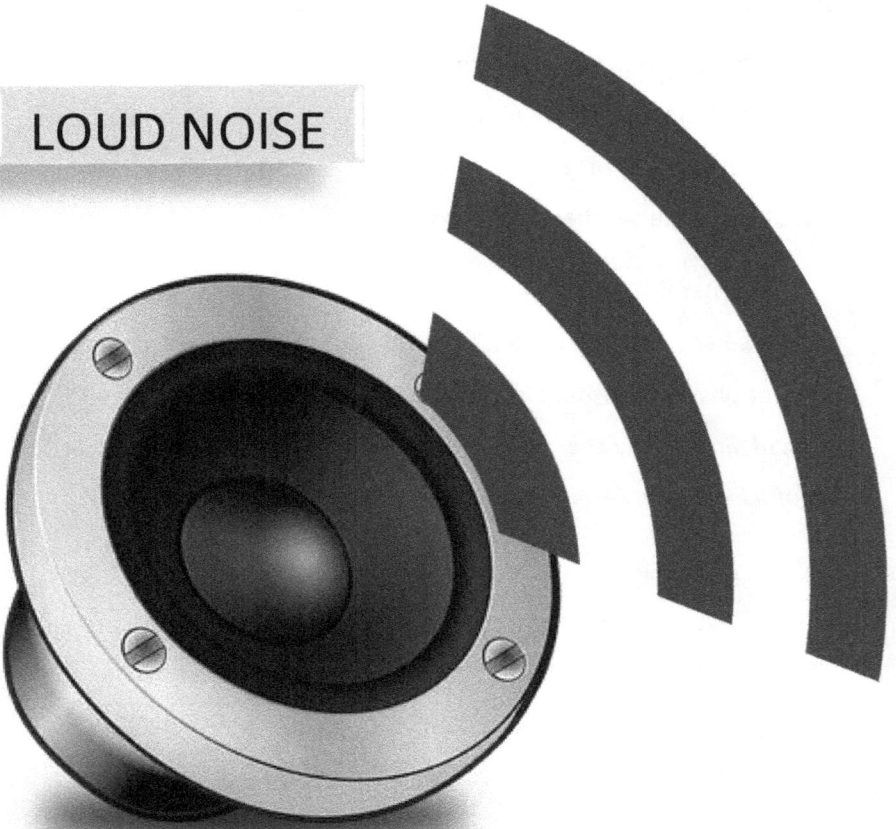

LOUD NOISE

According to a 2000 study from *Noise Health*, "noise causes the release of different stress hormones (59). A separate study from 2016, found increased cortisol levels following a loud noise at night during while subjects were sleeping (22).

COMMUTE/TRAFFIC

In a 1988 study from the International Archives of Occupational and Environmental Health found that *"available date indicate commuting to be a stress factor not only because of transport modes, but also by its interference with living and working conditions: namely, reduction of time available for discretionary leisure activities and increased absenteeism at workplace (8)."*

A 2006 study looked at the stress and cortisol levels of 208 rail commuters traveling from New Jersey to Manhattan. Salivary cortisol levels were tested directly upon arrival. The subjects were also given a proofreading stress test followed by a perceived stress evaluation. The researchers found that longer commutes had a significant association with higher cortisol levels, greater stress levels, and negative performances on the proofreading test (18).

SMOKING

"Just 2 cigarettes a day leads to consistent activation of the HPA axis, attenuating the responsiveness of the HPA axis to psychological stress (51)"

Per a 2006 study from the International Journal of Psychophysiology, "smokers also often have low grade systemic inflammation and decreased glucocorticoid sensitivity. These "may be causally related to disinhibition of inflammatory processes and thereby further stimulate adverse health outcomes, such as airway inflammation or atherosclerosis smokers often present with low-grade systemic inflammation (51)."

PHYSICAL PAIN

Baliki M, Geha P, Apkarian A, Chialvo D. **Beyond feeling: chronic back pain hurts the brain, disrupting the default mode network dynamics.** *Journal of Neuroscience.* 28(6); Pp 1398-1403. 2008.

- Researchers used MRI imaging of the brain to investigate the correlation between subjects suffering from low back pain and their ability to perform **simple visual tasks**.

- The **subjects with low back pain had constant activity in their front area of their brain associated with emotion.**

- **The researchers were concerned the nerves in this area of the brain may die off due to the over-activity, leading to shrinking of the brain.** This may lead to some of the cognitive impairments associated with chronic pain including depression, anxiety, and difficulty focusing (

Tagliazucchi E, Balenzuela P, Fraimain D, Chialvo D. **Brain resting state is disrupted in chronic back pain patients.** *Neuroscience Letters.* 485(1); Pp 26-31. 2010.

- Researchers compared the brain function of 12 chronic back patients with the functioning of 20 healthy controls.

- The researchers found alterations in the corticol regions of the brain known as **default mode network**, even during periods of rest.

- They concluded that chronic back pain may affect this area of the brain, potentially leading to cognitive and behavioral impairments

POSTURE

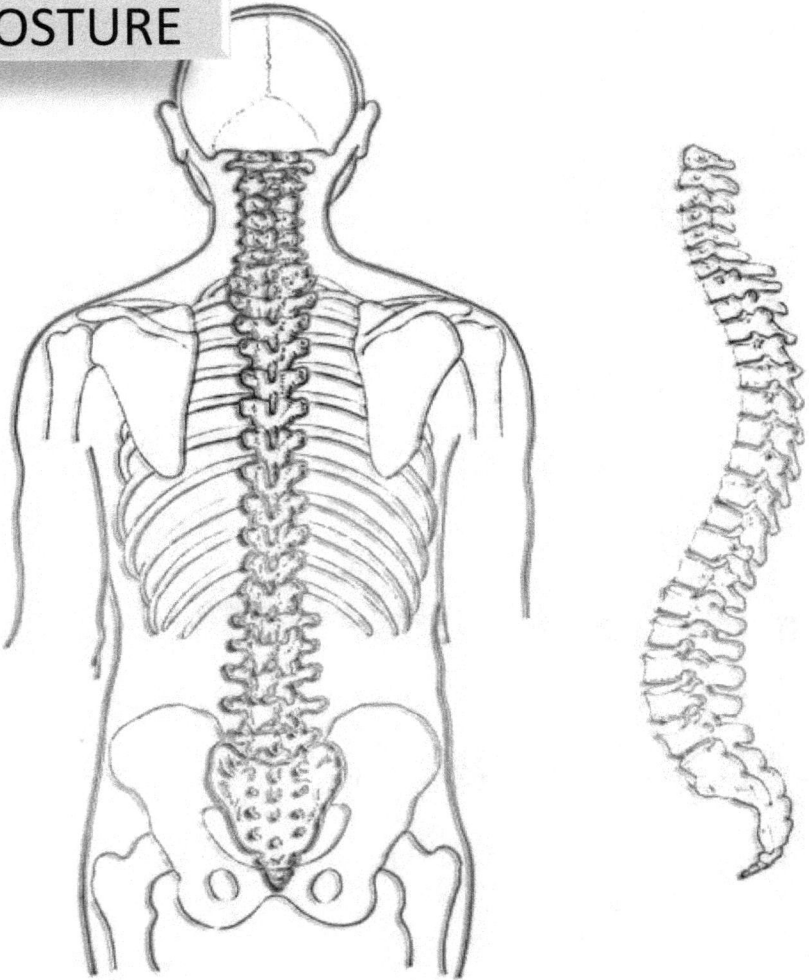

A 2010 study from *Psychological Science Online* titled

Power Posing: Brief nonverbal displays affect neuroendocrine

levels and risk tolerance found that by simply displaying/holding dominant postures for roughly one to two minutes, subjects could increase testosterone levels by nearly 20% (6).

Other studies have shown similar associations between testosterone and posture (1,43).

A 1982 study from *Motivation and Emotion* stated "*By simply changing physical posture, an individual prepares his or her mental and physiological systems to endure difficult and stressful situations, and perhaps to actually improve confidence and performance in situations such as interviewing for jobs, speaking in public, disagreeing with a boss, or taking potentially profitable risks (50).*"

According to a 1993 study from the *Journal of Personality and Social Psychology* found that hunched forward postures elicited greater feelings of depression (65) while a separate study from 1998 found that tilting the head upward produced a greater sense of pride (66).

Finally, a 2016 study from *Frontiers in Aging Neuroscience* found a link between postural alignment and cognitive function in older adults. The researchers found that those with forward head postures did worse on memory tasks. The paper also expressed that "*unobtrusive contraction of the "smile muscle" can increase enjoyment (7).*"

HORMONAL IMBALANCES

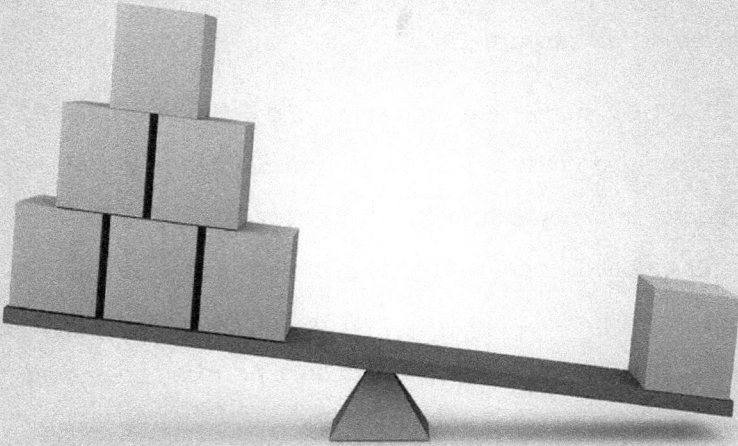

Research has shown that diabetics who survived the 2011 tsunami in Japan had decreased glycemic control and impaired glucose tolerance. The researchers theorized the blood sugar regulation had been altered due to the posttraumatic stress that resulted from the tsunami.

High cortisol can lead to excessive release of glucose into the bloodstream leading to alterations in blood sugar regulation. Too much glucose in the bloodstream increases the potential for glycation, an inflammatory inducing process in which sugars in the blood stream combine with proteins and fats forming AGEs, Advanced Glycation End-Products.

High cortisol can lead to estrogen dominance as cortisol competes with progesterone at the progesterone receptors. This can lead to an increase in estradiol as well as sex hormone binding globulin which in turn can decrease testosterone.

Low levels of testosterone have been linked to low levels of thyroid function (55). Chronically high cortisol can also influence both the production of thyroid stimulating hormone as well as the conversion of inactive T4 to active T3. Cortisol can also impact the responsiveness of tissue to thyroid hormone.

EXCESSIVE ENDURANCE TRAINING

"Research shows long distance cardiovascular exercise can decrease testosterone and raise cortisol (56)"

A study from the *Journal of Sport Sciences and Medicine* expressed that *"a link has been hypothesized between increased oxidative stress and plasma stress hormones (12)"* The study further states that "elevated cortisol levels might deplete cellular glutathione, which is an important substrate in antioxidant defense (12).

The study concluded that *"skiers with the lowest nutrient intake during the competition were the ones who showed greater cell damage and lower antioxidant enzyme activity and cortisol levels, which may impair performance and cause injuries and accidents (12)"*

A second study, this one from the 2011 *Psychoneuroendocrinology* journal looked at 304 endurance athletes and found that the higher the training volume, the higher the cortisol levels and lower the testosterone in those athletes (56).

JAW/HIP

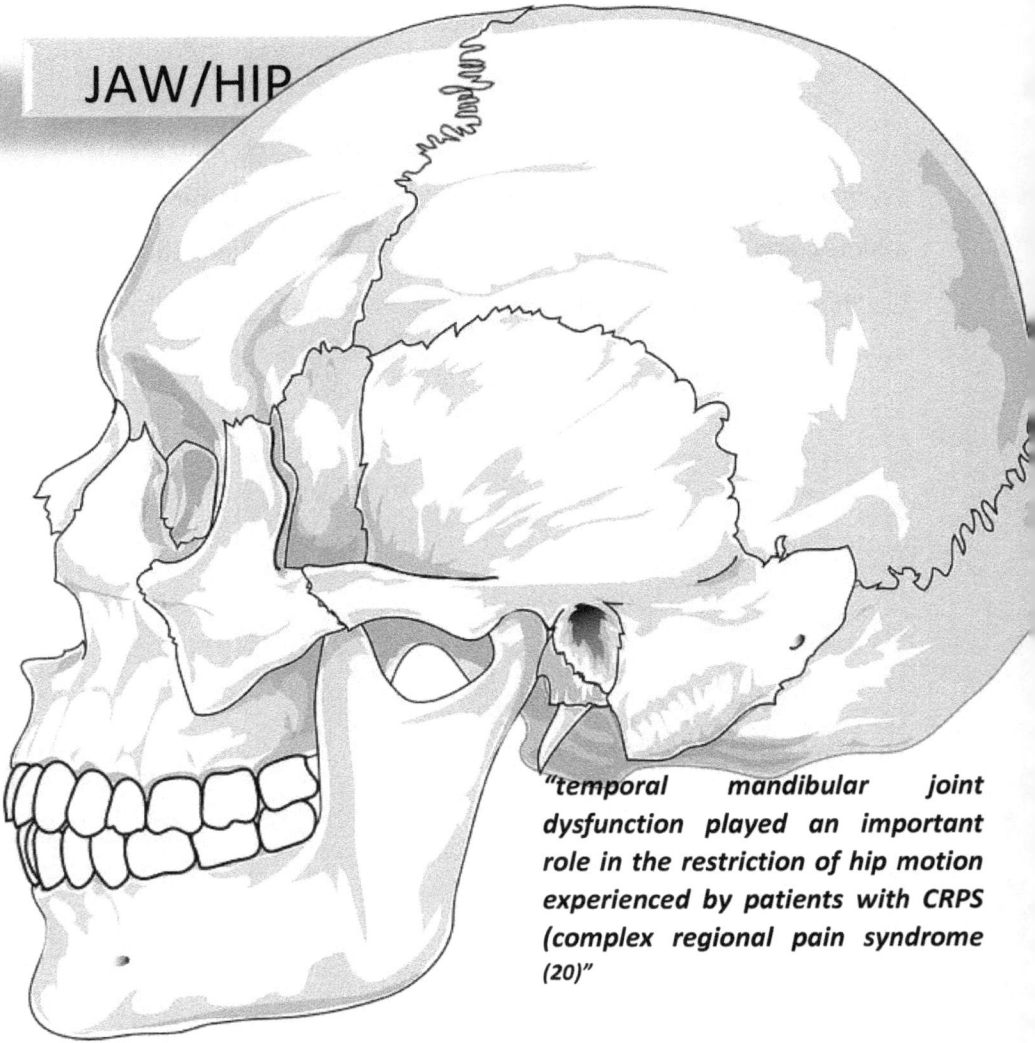

"temporal mandibular joint dysfunction played an important role in the restriction of hip motion experienced by patients with CRPS (complex regional pain syndrome (20)"

According to a 2012 article titled **Connecting Tension in The Hips and Jaw**, *"One study on the effects on hip pain of myofascial release massage techniques performed at the jaw,* *strongly suggest that clenching the jaw increased hip pain while massage therapy on the jaw relieved it (23)."*

That same article expresses that if your right side of the jaw is more clenched than the left, the right-side hip muscles are often more tense than those on the left or vice versa (23).

A 2008 study from *SOTO* found that *"the emerging evidence is indeed finding that relationships exist between ascending and descending contributions to CMD/TMD and postural dysfunctions (4).* This study also pointed out something quite interesting in that an *"anterior cruciate ligament injury may have an effect on muscle activity of head, neck and trunk muscles (4)."*

In 2007 Sakaguchi et al found that "there appears to be a cause and effect relationship between external derangement-type TMD and sacroiliac sprain (52)." The researchers found that subjects habitual bite affected body postures.

Per a 2009 study from the *Journal of Manipulative and Physiological Therapeutics* jaw joint dysfunction played a significant role in hip mobility indicating *"a connectedness between these two regions of the body (20)."*

Lucerini F, Ponzio E, Di Palma M, Galati C, Federici A, Barbadoro P, D'errico M, Prospero E, Amborgini P, Cuppini R, Lattanzi D, Minielli A. **High cardiorespiratory fitness is negatively associated with daily cortisol output in healthy aging men.** PLOS ONE. 10(11); Pp 1-15, 2015.

29 subjects

Day 1:

Rockport walking test for fitness assessment; High Fit or Low Fit

- 6 salivary cortisol samples were taken

Day 2: Color Word Interference Stroop Test (3 mins) + 2 min Mental Arithmetic task counting backwards from 2083 in 17 steps as quickly as possible

- Cortisol taken 10 min before, 5 min, 20 min, and 60 mins after.

In the present study, possible associations between aerobic fitness and the cortisol response to acute mental stress were evaluated in elderly men, with the results indicating that high fit subjects tend to exhibit a larger response, and steeper cortisol decline during recovery compared to their low fit counterparts

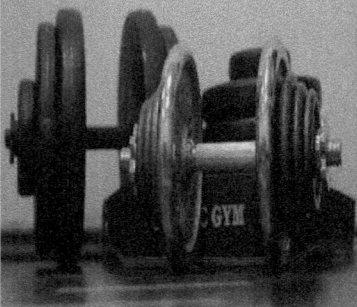

ACTIVITY FITNESS LEVELS AND STRESS CONT...

High Fit vs Low Fit Cortisol Levels

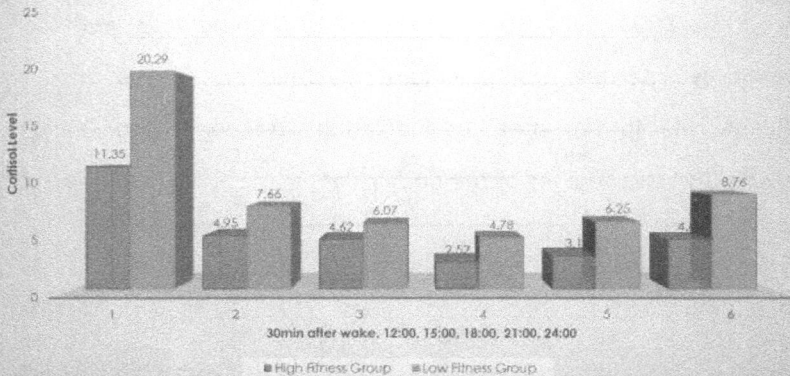

Cortisol Level

11.35, 20.29, 4.95, 7.66, 4.62, 6.07, 2.57, 4.78, 6.25, 8.76

30min after wake, 12:00, 15:00, 18:00, 21:00, 24:00

■ High Fitness Group   ■ Low Fitness Group

CHAPTER 2: HOW STRESS AFFECTS THE BODY

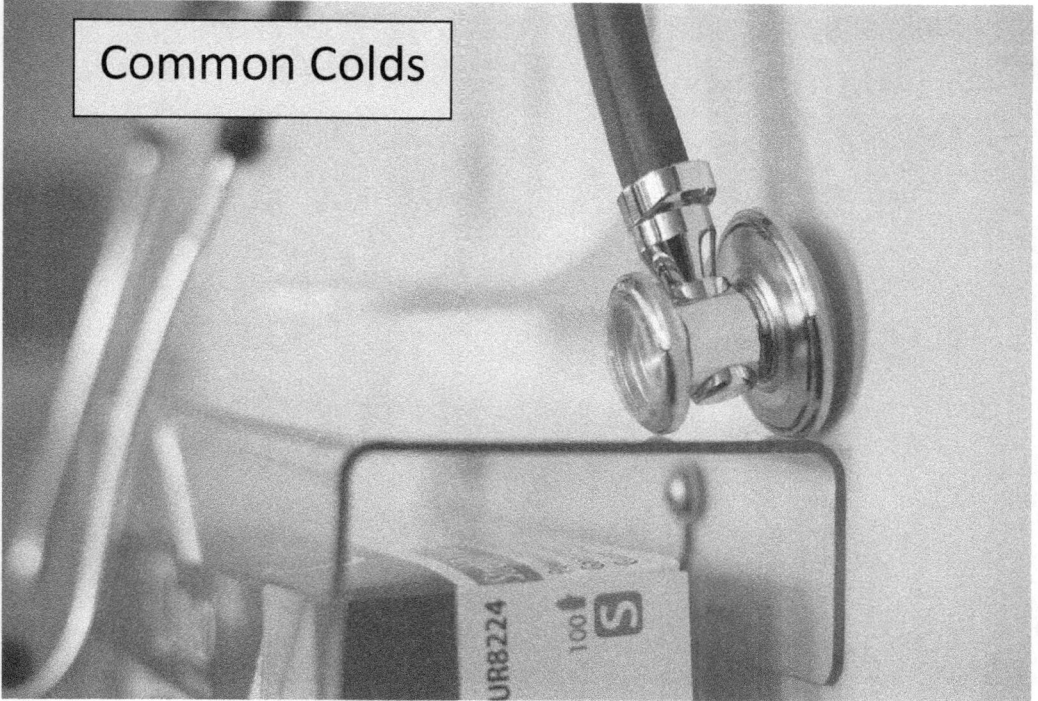

Common Colds

A 2012 study out of Carnegie Melon found that *"those subjects with altered or decreased ability to manage the inflammatory response to the virus had greater susceptibility toward developing the cold than those with healthy inflammatory responses (3)."*

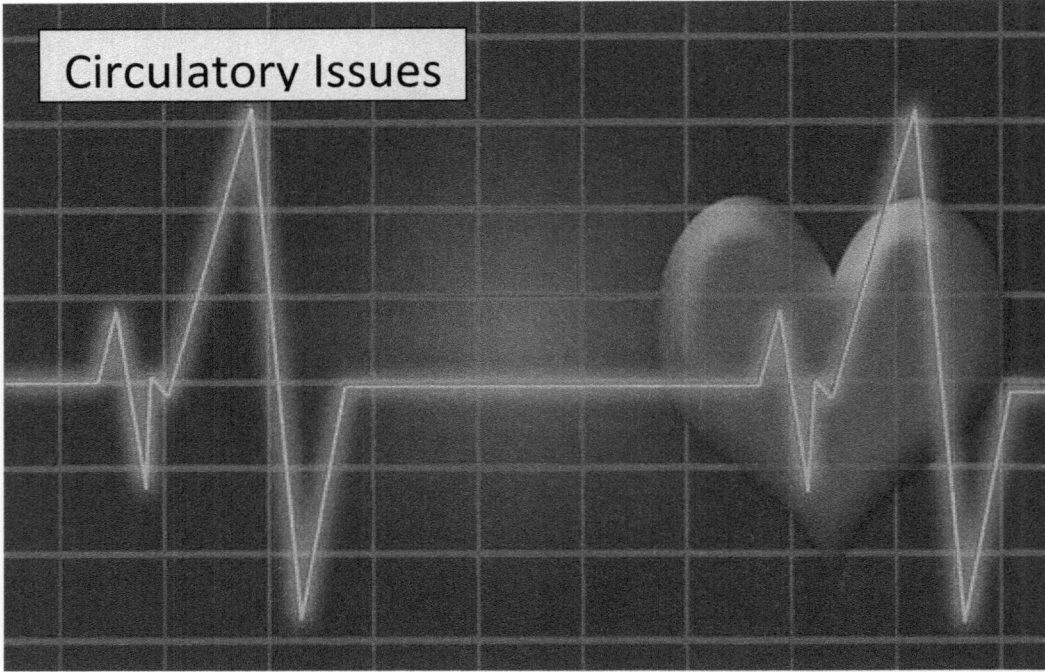

Circulatory Issues

Did you know that 22.4% out of 838 Raynaud's attacks were reported to be caused by emotional stress (6)? A study from the British Medical Journal found that *"In Raynaud's disease about one third of the vasospastic attacks were associated with tachycardia and increased stress ratings with declines in ambient temperature (6)."*

Decreased Flexibility

"When physical or mental fatigue occur, flexibility is reduced (13)"

Think vertical column muscle groups here. Hip flexors, hamstrings, sternocleidomastoid (neck muscles) etc. According to Thieme, *"Muscle control, of course, does not take place exclusively at the level of the spinal cord and muscle. Presumably, only the reflex processes used in the various stretching techniques occur at this level, which is subordinate to various brain centers that exert activating or inhibiting effects (13)."*

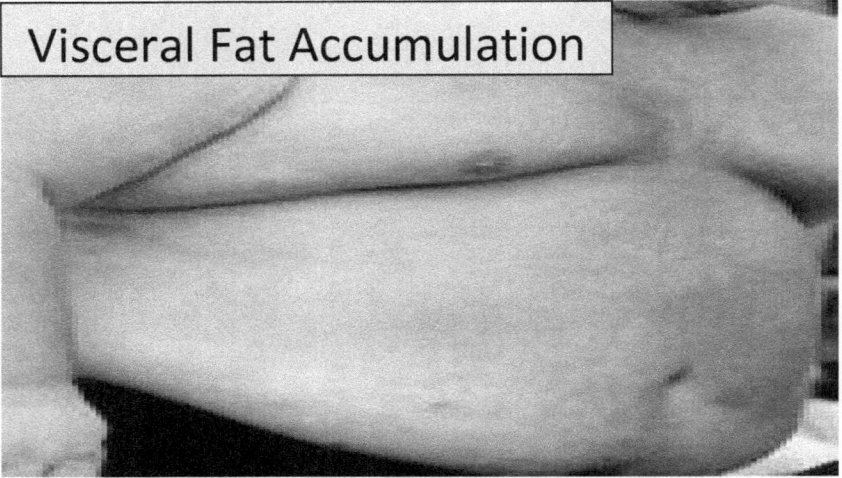

Visceral Fat Accumulation

According to a 2003 study from *Panminerva Medica* *"it is well known that central obesity is associated with elevated cortisol secretion (4)."* The study continues *"cumulative exposure to cortisol could contribute to increased visceral fat (4)".* Lastly the authors expressed *"psychosocial and economic handicaps, depressive and anxiety traits, alcohol and smoking can act as a stressor and thus activate the HPA axis. Many of these conditions are associated with visceral fat accumulation (4)."*

Muscle Tightness

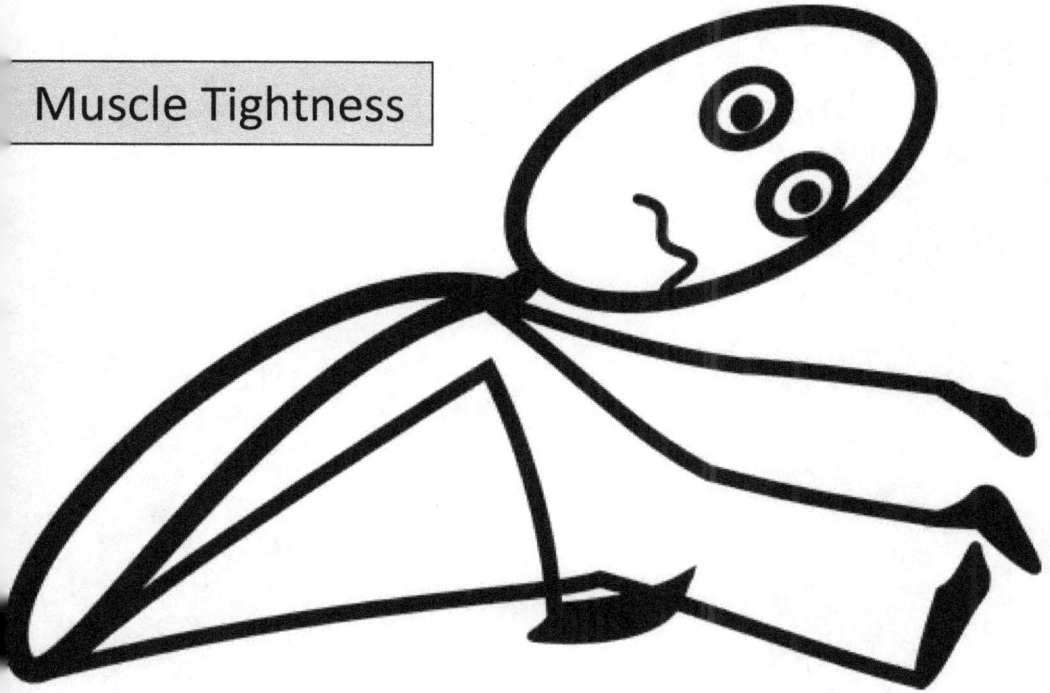

A 2014 article titled ***Stretching Your Stress Out- Meet Your Psoas*** expresses *"the deeper part of the body stores stress as well; the hips. The psoas is the main muscle of the "fight or flight" response of the body. When you are startled, your psoas contracts, when you have mental or emotional stress, the psoas will respond by tightening (2)."*

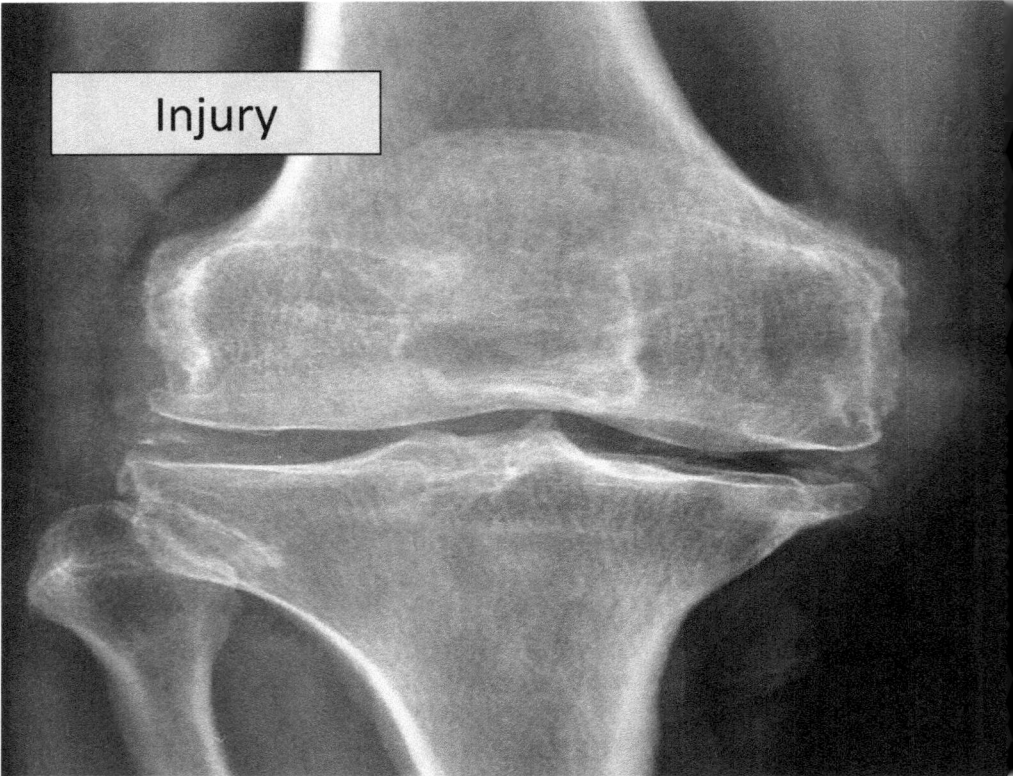

Injury

In an eye opening 2012 article titled **How the Adrenals Affect Muscles, Ligaments, and Joints in The Body**, the author expresses that *"an inguinal hernia is a sign of adrenal fatigue. The inguinal ligament runs from the lateral edge of the anterior superior iliac spine (ASIS) to the pubic bone. This ligament supports the region around the groin between the abdomen and the thigh, also preventing an inguinal hernia or a protrusion of part of the intestine into the muscle or the groin (11)."*

The article continues *"Muscle organ correlations were discovered by Dr. Goodhart in the 1960's. He found that there are predicable muscle imbalances when organs are in stress. In the case of the adrenal glands one of the primary muscles involved is the Sartorius, a major pelvic as well as medial knee stabilizer (Sartorius is the longest muscle in the human body, it runs down the length of the thigh). This is why so many people including athletes injure their knees when they are under stress. There was a pre-existing imbalance from the adrenals that caused an improper or inadequate response of the Sartorius muscle. So, the demand on muscle exceeded its threshold to handle it and this results in an injury (11)."*

Finally, the article expresses *"the direct connection to the low back from stress is that the Sartorius imbalance in the front of the thigh has an impact on the sacroiliac joint integrity on the posterior side of the pelvis (11)."*

A separate article, this one from the 2015 edition the *National Scholastic Athletics Foundation* carries the torch further in describing the connection between hip flexor tightness and how it leads to chronic injuries in runners. The author states *"proper running posture consists of a slight forward lean and anterior pelvic tilt. An excessive forward lean while running suggests that the posterior chain muscles (hamstrings, gluteals, and erector spinae) are not strong enough, which increases strain on the hamstrings and back during the running action. A posture that is too upright indicates exaggerated pelvic anterior-posterior tilt, meaning the gluteals and abdominals do not have enough strength to control the pelvis adequately during landing. An excessive anterior pelvic tilt increases the ground impact through the lumbar and sacroiliac joints and forces the knee to internally rotate, which in turn may increase the pronating forces on the ankle. An exaggerated pelvic AP tilt can have negative effects on other muscles. The most common side effect is a tightened piriformis and hip adductor complex. The piriformis is a deep muscle and is the most powerful external rotator of the hip. A tight piriformis can lead to problems with the knees and piriformis syndrome. Piriformis syndrome occurs when the piriformis irritates the sciatic nerve and causes a deep shooting pain from the buttocks down the back of the leg (8)."*

Tight hip flexors can affect head posture *"When the hip flexors are excessively tight they cause exaggerated pelvic anterior tilt. The lumbar spine becomes excessively arched and the thoracic spine develops a kyphotic alignment, which can lead to forward head posture (8)."*

Thermoregulation

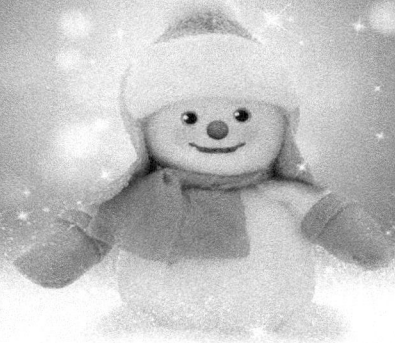

Did you know that a 2014 study from the *Clinical Journal of Pain* found that the same areas of the brain that are responsible for regulation of pain are also responsible for regulation of temperature? The authors express that *"the challenge of maintaining normal body temperatures in the face of acute cold or of **initiating adaptive thermogenesis in response to chronic stress** may be compromised by conditions that are comorbid with fibromyalgia (9)."*

The study further expresses that *"patients with fibromyalgia often report physical or emotional trauma prior to the onset of their condition, and **stress exacerbates their symptoms** (9)."*

Stomach Acid

"*Stress and cortisol can have a negative impact stomach acid levels, which can open the door to a whole host of health issues (12)*"

Decreased Wound Healing

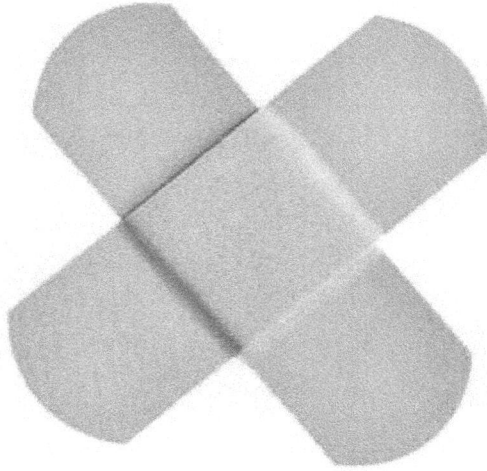

A 2004 study from the journal *Psychoneuroendocrinology* looked at perceived stress and cortisol levels and how these impacted the rate of wound healing. The researchers found that the higher the cortisol levels, the longer it took wounds to heal (5).

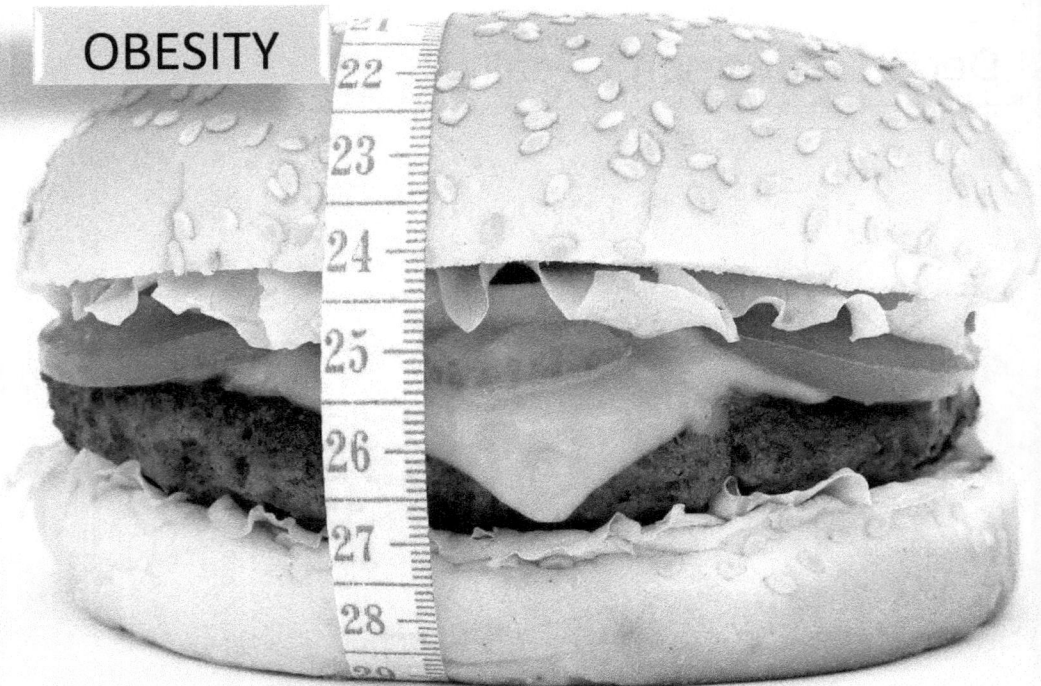

OBESITY

Per a 2009 study that followed nationally representative cohort of US adults for over 9 years, "*psychosocial stress was associated with greater weight gain among both men and women with higher baseline body mass indexes if they experienced job related demands, had difficulty paying bills, or had depression or generalized anxiety disorder (1).*"

Cancer

A 2010 study from *Future Oncology* stated that ""*Clinical and epidemiological studies over the last 30 years have identified psychosocial factors including stress, chronic depression and lack of social support as risk factors for cancer progression (10)*."

Etc...

Steptoe A, Kivimaki M. **Stress and cardiovascular disease: an update in current knowledge.** *Annu Rev Publ Health.* 34; Pp 337. 2013.

*Frequent HPA activation and increased cortisol secretion are proposed as being etiological in the development of several chronic conditions that become manifest in the older population, including **cardiovascular disease***

Comjis H, Gerritsen L, Penninx B, Bremmer M, Deeg D, Geerlings M. **The association between serum cortisol and cognitive decline in older persons.** *American Journal of Geriatric Psychiatry.* 18(1); Pp 42-50. 2010.

*A growing body of evidence from cross sectional and prospective studies has shown that **high levels of cortisol secretion correlate with poor cognitive outcomes in older adults:** men and women in the top quartile of baseline cortisol had a larger decline in cognitive functions measured over a 7 year follow up period*

Belvederi Murri M, Pariante C, Mondelli V, Masotti M, Atti A, Mellacqua Z, et al. **HPA axis and aging in depression: systematic review and meta-analysis.** *Psychoneuroendocrinology.* 41; Pp 46-62. 2014.

*Chronically elevated cortisol levels are associated with the development of **depression***

Holanda C, Guerra R, Nobrega P, Costa H, Piuvezam M, Maciel A. **Salivary cortisol and frailty syndrome in elderly residents of long-stay institutions: a cross-sectional study.** *Archives of Gerontology and Geriatrics.* 54(2); Pp 146-151. 2012.

*High cortisol levels can lead to **frailty.***

Marcell T. **Sarcopenia: causes, consequences, and preventions.** *The Journals of Gerontology Series A: Biological Sciences and Medical Sciences.* 58(10); Pp 911-916. 2003.

Cortisol is a catabolic hormone that stimulates **degradation and inhibits the synthesis of muscle proteins**, thus causing sarcopenia

Peeters G, can Schoor N, Visser M, Knol D, Eekhoff E, de Ronde W, et al. **Relationship between cortisol and physical performance in older persons.** *Clinical Endocrinology.* 67(3); Pp 398-406. 2007.

Chronically elevated levels of cortisol production may thus **affect VOm2max** due to the gradual loss of metabolically active muscle mass. In support of the latter view, alterations in circadian cortisol secretion have been found to be associate with several physical conditions that become manifest at an older age: higher cortisol levels have been associated with a **worse physical performance** in healthy older adults

Franz C, Obrien R, Hauger R, Mendoza S, Panizzon M, Prom-Wormley E, et al. **Cross sectional and 35-year longitudinal assessment of salivary cortisol and cognitive functioning: the Vietnam Era twin study of aging.** *Psychoneuroendorcinology.* 36(7); Pp 1040-1052. 2011.

Higher levels of cortisol output predicted poorer performance in **executive functions and visual spatial memory**

Bull C, Christensen H, Fenech M. **Cortisol is not associated with telomere shortening or chromosomal instability in human lymphocytes cultured under low and high folate conditions.** *PLoS One.* 10(3); e0119367. 2015.

*"Psychological stress is one factor that has been associated with accelerated telomere shortening in lymphocytes or leukocytes. Numerous studies have shown that chronically stressed individuals have significantly **shorter telomeres than those with lower perceived and/or actual stress**, and that stress and adversity **experienced during childhood results in shortened telomeres and chromosomal damage (micronuclei) in adults"***

CHAPTER 3: STRESS STRATEGIES

7
Characteristics
of Highly
Resilient
People

1. PRESENCE DE ESPRIT

Everly G. McCormack D. Strouse D. Seven characteristics of highly resilient people: Insights from Navy SEALs to the "Greatest Generation". International Journal of Emergency Mental Health. 14(2): Pp 137-143. 2012.

"or calm, innovative, non-dogmatic thinking. Having the presence of mind to think in a calm, rational manner, especially under stress is rare. The ability to see old problems from a new perspective is key to overcoming hindrances that stifle others."

"The essential focus is not concentrating on what is wrong, per se, but rather, having defined the problem, the focus is on finding a novel solution. "

2. DECISIVE ACTION

Everly G. McCormack D. Strouse D. Seven characteristics of highly resilient people: Insights from Navy SEALs to the "Greatest Generation". International Journal of Emergency Mental Health. 14(2): Pp 137-143. 2012.

"Once a decision has been reached, it is essential to act decisively. "The hesitancy that typifies non-resilient decision-making is often the fear of making a mistake, or failing. The corollary to decisive action, however is the necessity to take responsibility for one's actions. Taking responsibility is sometimes difficult, especially if the action leads to an undesirable outcome. However, highly resilient people are often the first to take responsibility because they see that as the first step toward resolution and subsequent success"

3. TENACITY

Everly G, McCormack D, Strouse D. Seven characteristics of highly resilient people: Insights from Navy SEALs to the "Greatest Generation". International Journal of Emergency Mental Health. 14(2): Pp 137-143. 2012.

"Great American success stories are replete with the theme of tenacity. In many cases it was not the genius that predicted success, it was the tenacity. Thomas Edison light bulb story. "it required over 6000 failed experiments to arrive at the right combination.""

4. INTERPERSONAL CONNECTEDNESS AND SUPPORT

Everly G, McCormack D, Strouse D. Seven characteristics of highly resilient people: Insights from Navy SEALs to the "Greatest Generation". International Journal of Emergency Mental Health. 14(2): Pp 137-143. 2012.

"may be the single most powerful predictor of human resilience. What characteristics are likely to engender the support of others? We believe amongst the most compelling is integrity."

5. INTEGRITY

Everly G, McCormack D, Strouse D. Seven characteristics of highly resilient people: Insights from Navy SEALs to the "Greatest Generation". International Journal of Emergency Mental Health. 14(2): Pp 137-143. 2012.

"doing that which is right. It is considering not only what is good for you, but what is good for others as well. Integrity engenders trust"

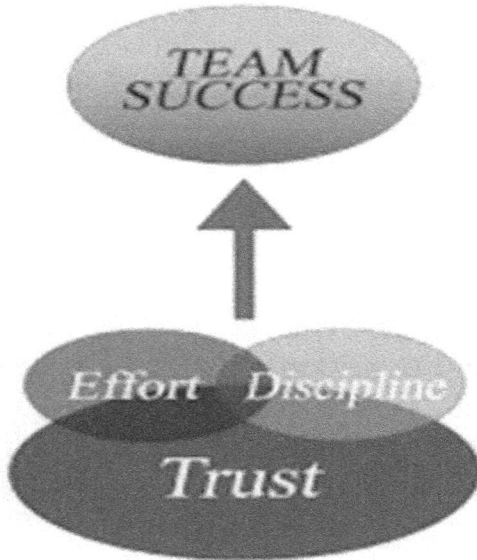

6. SELF-DISCIPLINE AND SELF-CONTROL

Everly G, McCormack D, Strouse D. Seven characteristics of highly resilient people: Insights from Navy SEALs to the "Greatest Generation". International Journal of Emergency Mental Health. 14(2): Pp 137-143. 2012.

"Perhaps the single most dangerous action one can take is the impulsive action. Road rage, airline rage, certain types of gambling and domestic violence may be related to the inability to practice self-control. On the other hand, we know certain health promoting behaviors, such as relaxation training, physical exercise, and practicing good nutrition require a certain self-discipline that many simply find too challenging to practice consistently."

7. OPTIMISM AND POSITIVE THINKING

Everly G, McCormack D, Strouse D. Seven characteristics of highly resilient people: Insights from Navy SEALs to the "Greatest Generation". International Journal of Emergency Mental Health. 14(2): Pp 137-143. 2012.

"Optimism is the tendency to expect the best outcome. Optimistic people are more perseverant and resilient than are pessimists. Optimistic people tend to be more task-oriented and committed to success than are pessimistic people. Optimistic people appear to tolerate adversity to a greater extent than do pessimists.

Recent research suggest there may be two types of optimism: passive and active. Passive optimism consists of hoping things will turn out well in the future. Active optimism is acting in a manner to increase the likelihood that things will indeed turn out well in the future."

7. OPTIMISM AND POSITIVE THINKING CONT......

Everly G. McCormack D. Strouse D. Seven characteristics of highly resilient people: Insights from Navy SEALs to the "Greatest Generation". International Journal of Emergency Mental Health. 14(2): Pp 137-143. 2012.

"A common characteristic of a Navy SEAL is the presence of a strong positive mental attitude which expects success. Success is a way of life for SEALs. It must be. Success does not happen by chance; from the SEAL perspective, it exists because one makes it so.

Dr. Albert Bandura book Self-Efficacy: The exercise of control. Bandura defines the perception of self efficacy as the belief in one's own ability to exercise control in a meaningful and positive way. More specifically, self efficacy is the optimistic belief in one's ability to organize and execute the courses of action required to achieve necessary and desired goals"

CONCLUSION

Everly G. McCormack D. Strouse D. Seven characteristics of highly resilient people: Insights from Navy SEALs to the "Greatest Generation". International Journal of Emergency Mental Health. 14(2): Pp 137-143. 2012.

"Theory and controlled empirical investigations alike appear to converge on the conclusion that the response to any stressful event will be greatly influenced by the **appraisal of the situation, the ability to attach a constructive meaning to the experience,** the **ability to foresee an effective means of coping with the challenges of a given situation,** and the ability to ultimately incorporate the experience into some overarching belief system or schema."

ANTI-STRESS DIET/FOOD CHOICES

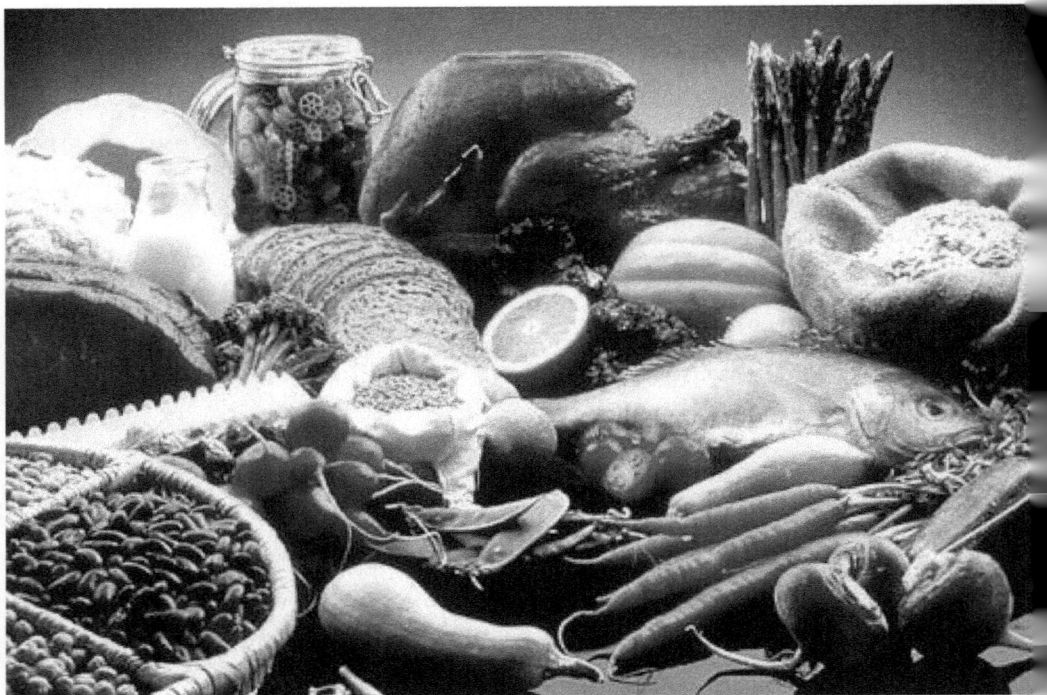

A 2017 study from *BMC Medicine* looked at the effects a higher quality fat, lower processed carb diet had on depression symptoms. The study had 67 subjects, half went on the Mediterranean Diet for 12 weeks, while the other half ate their normal diet for 12 weeks. After 12 weeks, the subjects eating the Mediterranean diet had significantly greater improvements in depression scores, leading the researchers to conclude that *"subjects with moderate to severe depression can improve their mood by eating a healthier diet (36)."*

Almonds

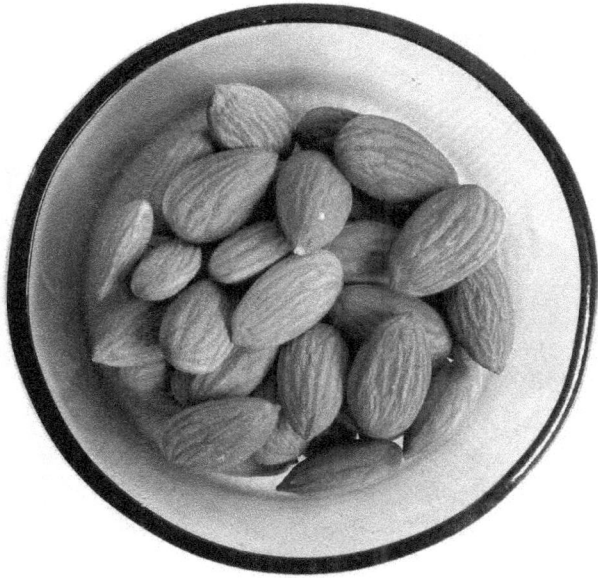

ALMONDS

- High levels of growth hormone promoting amino acid Arginine.
- Magnesium
- Manganese
- Phosphorus
- Iron
- Vitamin E
- Vitamin B2, B3, B9
- 6g protein/oz
- 3g fiber in 1oz
- About 90% of almond fat consists of mono- and polyunsaturated fatty acids
- Antioxidants: resveratrol, catechin, epicatechin, Quercitin
- Lower LDL while raising HDL

Asparagus

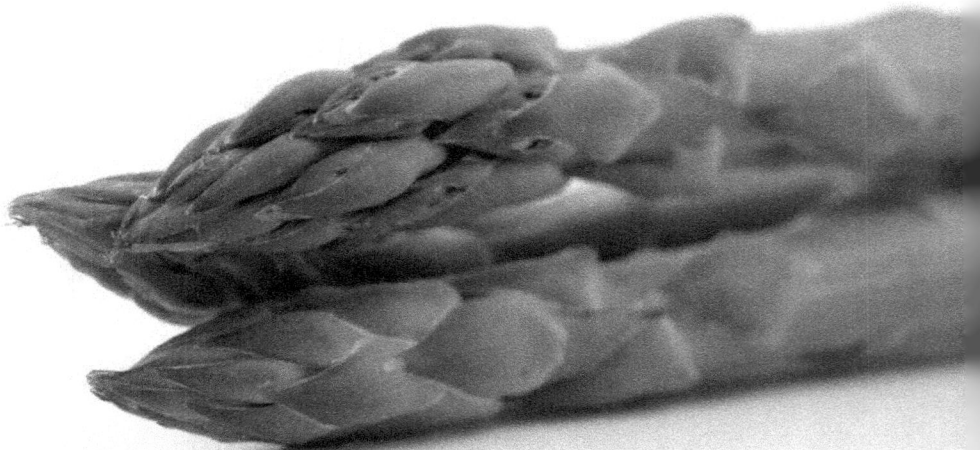

ASPARAGUS
- About 2-3 grams of prebiotic inulin per 3.5-ozserving.
- Asparagus has been shown to promote friendly bacteria in the gut and has been linked to the prevention of certain cancers
- High in folate, which is good for keeping calm

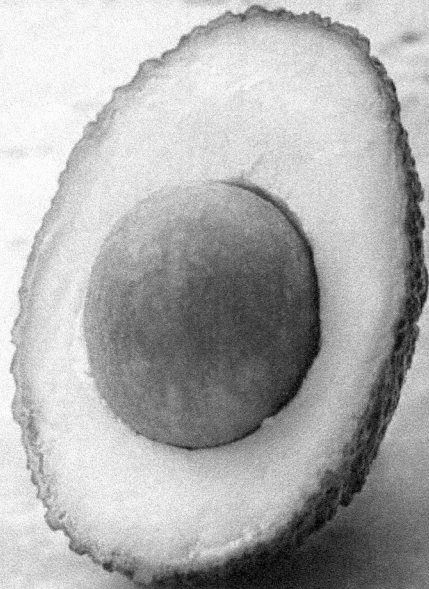

Avocado

AVOCADO

- 15g of quality fat, particularly oleic acid
- 4.5g fiber
- Rich in glutathione, a substance that specifically blocks intestinal absorption of certain fats that cause oxidative damage.
- Potassium, copper, and magnesium
- Vitamin C and E
- Vitamin B6 and B9
- Vitamin K1
- Also contain lutein, beta-carotene

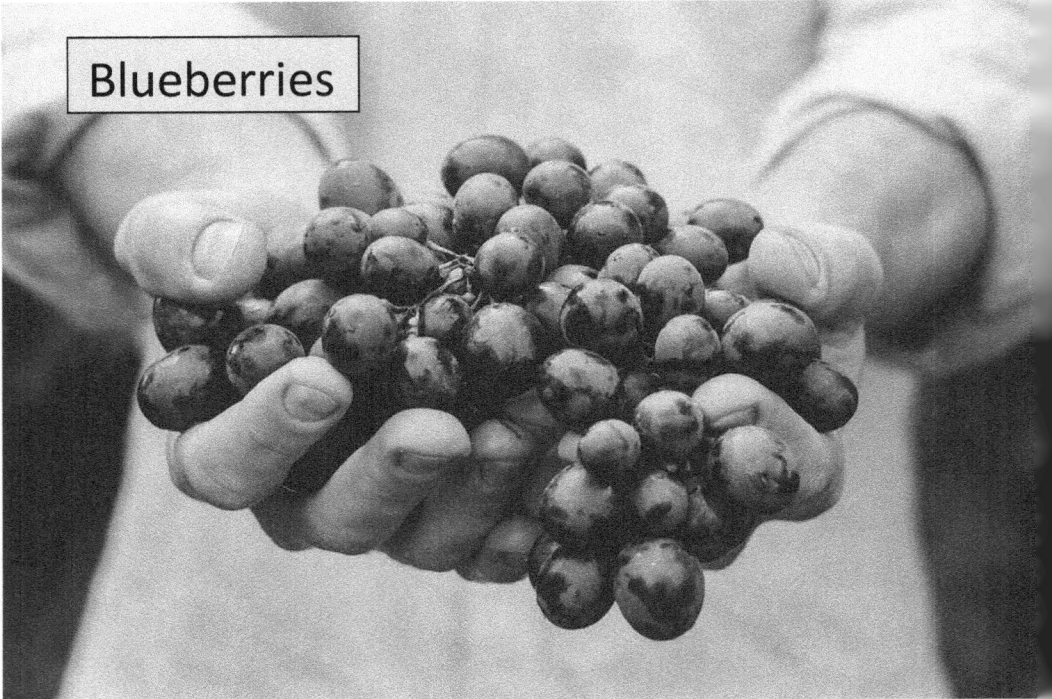

Blueberries

BLUEBERRIES

- ➢ 3.6g fiber per cup
- ➢ High in vitamin C, E, and K1
- ➢ Contains Manganese and Copper
- ➢ Contains flavanols Quercetin and Myricetin
- ➢ Have some of the highest levels of anthocyanin and have been linked to sharper cognition. German researchers tested this by asking 120 people to give a speech, then do hard math problems. Those who had eaten blueberries had lower blood pressure and lower levels of cortisol after the stressful situations.
- ➢ Blueberries have also been shown in studies to improve cognition and protect the brain.

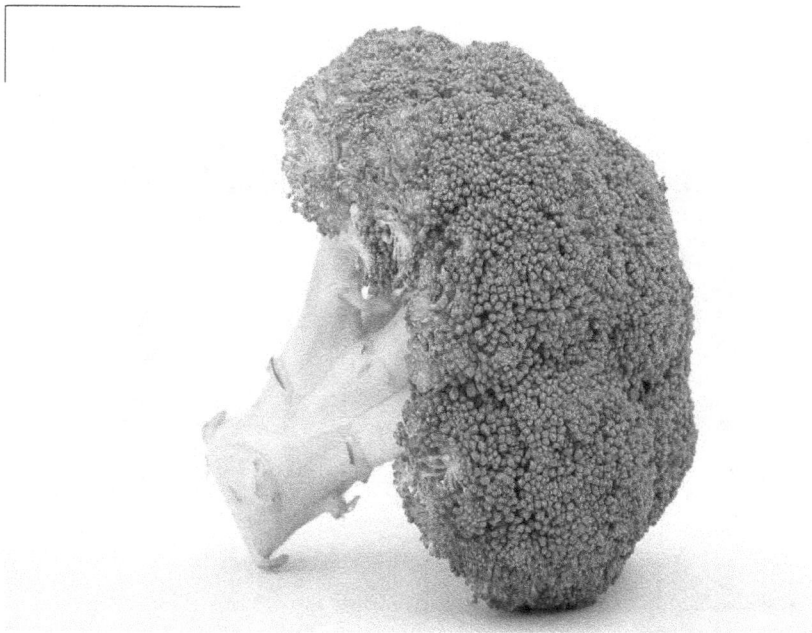

BROCCOLI

- ➤ 1 cup 2.3g fiber
- ➤ One of the highest vegetables for protein at 3g per cup
- ➤ Abundant in Potassium, Manganese, and Iron
- ➤ Contains the highest level of vitamin C (165% daily value)
- ➤ Vitamin K1 and folate
- ➤ Sulforaphane: may have protective effects against certain cancers
- ➤ Indole-3-carbinol: also, has protective effects
- ➤ Quercetin
- ➤ Lutein, zeaxanthin and beta-carotene

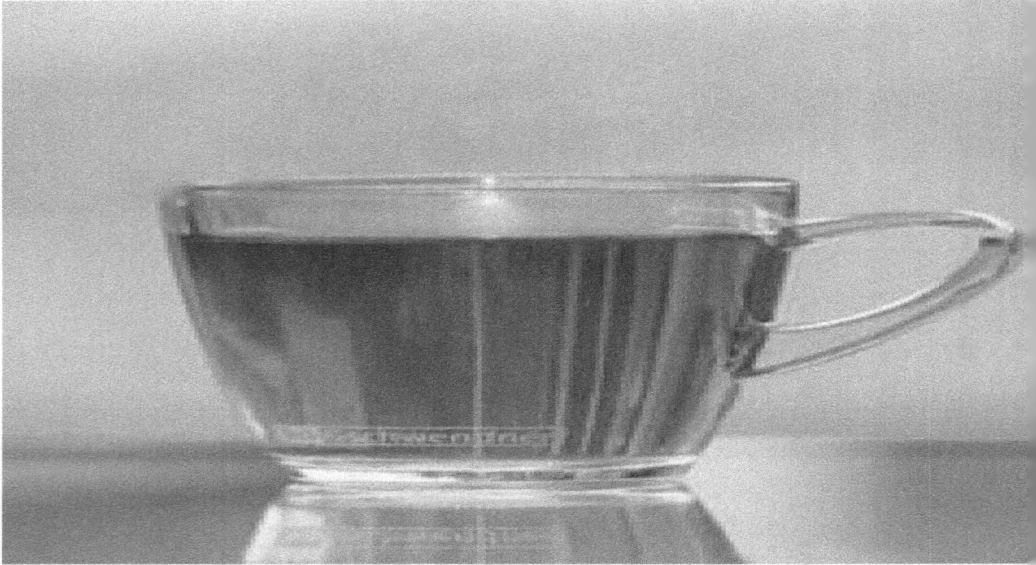

CHAMOMILE TEA

> ➤ University of Pennsylvania study tested chamomile supplements on 57 participants with generalized anxiety disorder for 8 weeks. They found a significant drop in anxiety after the 8 weeks

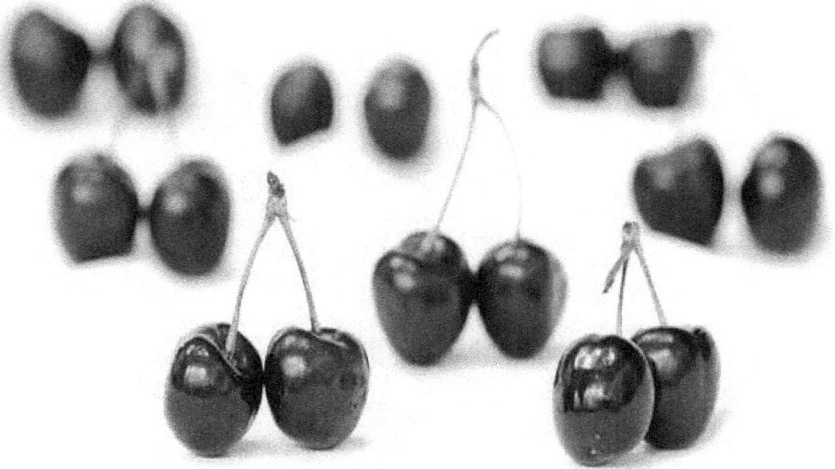

Cherries

CHERRIES

> A 2012 study from *Experimental Gerontology* gave 30 subjects extract from cherries broken into two separate servings per day for 5 days. The group consuming the cherry extract had **lower cortisol and higher serotonin levels** (30).

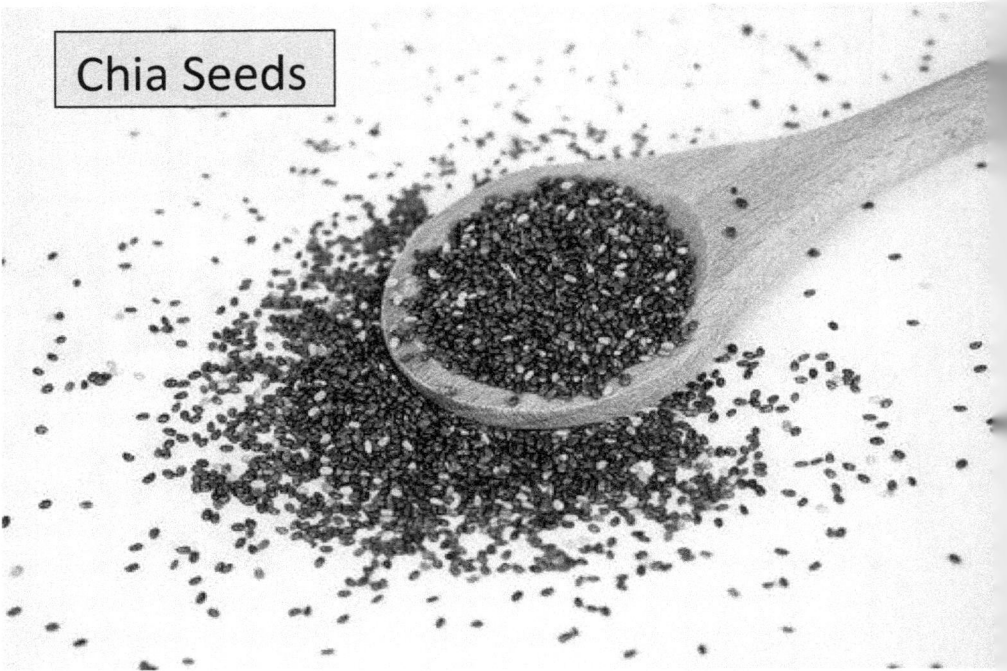

Chia Seeds

CHIA SEED

➢ **Roughly 75% of the fats are omega-3 fatty acid alpha linolenic acid (ALA)**

➢ **High in calcium, boron, magnesium, phosphorus, manganese, copper, and iron**

➢ **Has more omega 3 fatty acids than salmon**

➢ **11g of fiber per ounce**

➢ **Contains Quercetin, chlorogenic acid, caffeic acid, and antioxidant Kaempferol**

Cinnamon

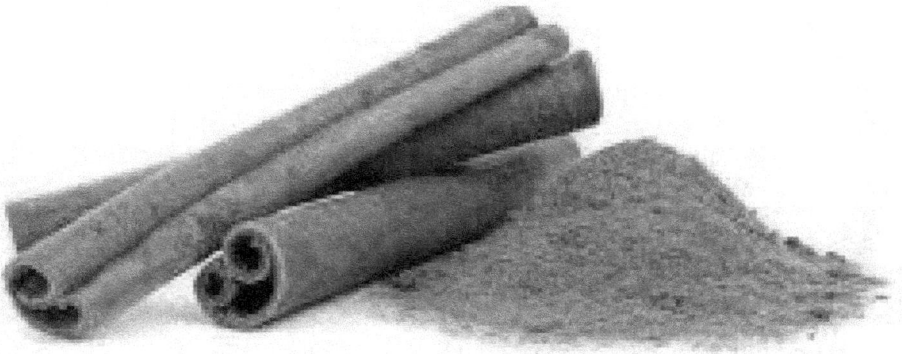

CINNAMON

- ➤ High in calcium, iron, fiber, and manganese
- ➤ 12-week study out of London found that 2g of cinnamon daily dropped A1C levels in diabetics by 7% as well as blood pressure
- ➤ Slows gastric emptying
- ➤ Increases insulin sensitivity
- ➤ One of the highest antioxidant capacities of any food source

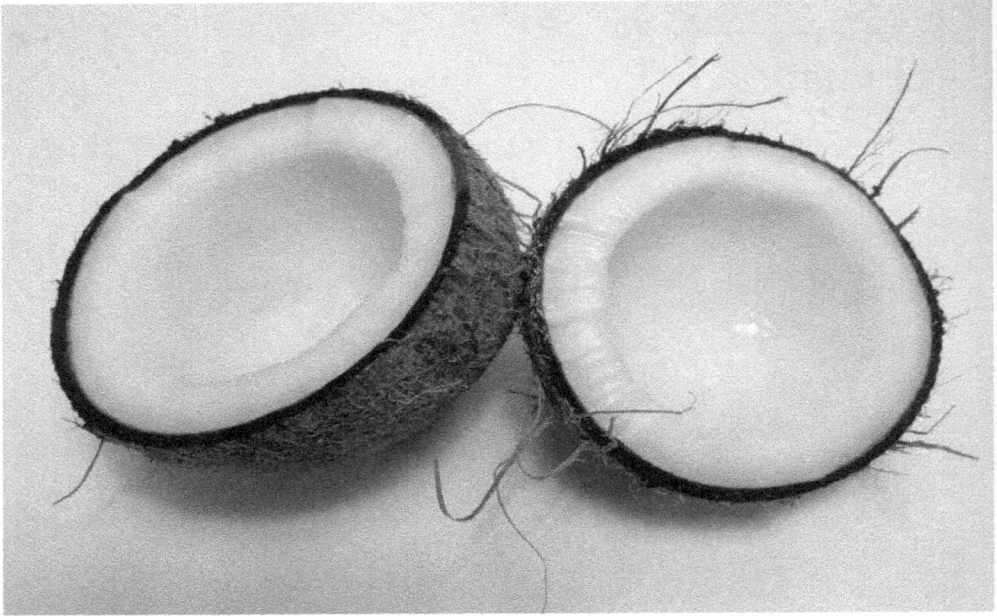

COCONUT

- ➢ High in MCT's which in turn increase lipid oxidation
- ➢ Reduces cholesterol, triglycerides, phospholipids, and LDL
- ➢ Improves digestion
- ➢ Contains lauric acid and monolaurin can kill harmful pathogens like bacteria, viruses, fungi, and parasites
- ➢ Breaks down kidney stones
- ➢ Can aid in recovering from food poisoning

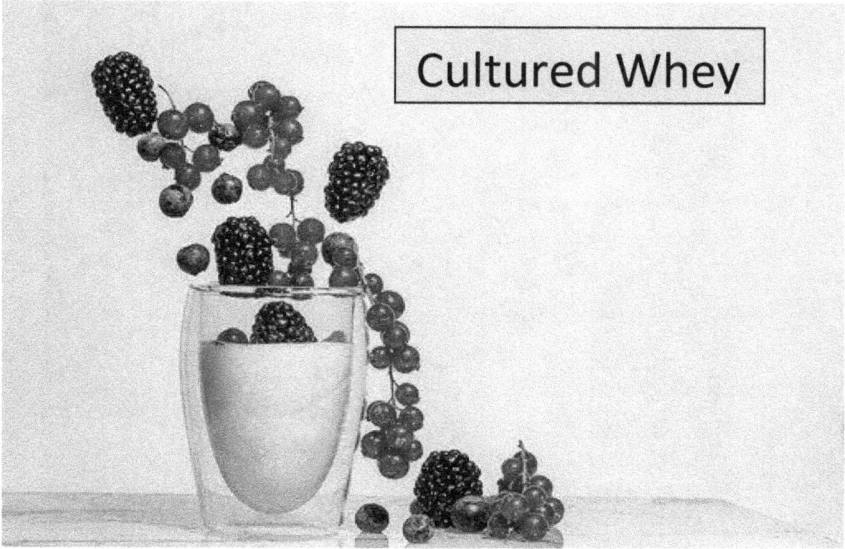

Cultured Whey

CULTURED WHEY/AMASAI

- ➢ Healing properties
- ➢ Stimulates intestinal peristalsis
- ➢ Generates intestinal flora
- ➢ Eliminates excess water retention
- ➢ Stimulates toxin elimination from the kidneys
- ➢ *E Coli was injected into raw milk, yogurt, and Amasai. The E coli flourished in the raw milk, yogurt killed it off in 4 days, while the Amasai killed it in 2 days."*

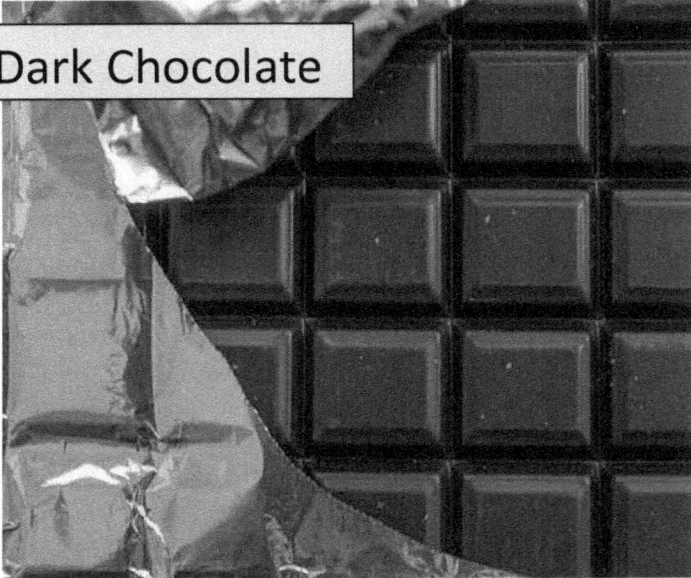

Dark Chocolate

DARK CHOCOLATE

A 2014 study in the *Journal of the American College of Cardiology* looked at the effects 125mg of dark chocolate had on stress levels, salivary cortisol and adrenaline. The researchers found that ingesting dark chocolate two hours before a stressful event buffered stress reactivity and decreased both cortisol and adrenaline levels. In the study the authors also pointed to a *"a 2009 study found that after eating dark chocolate every day for two weeks, people who rated themselves as highly stressed had lower levels of cortisol and catecholamines (81)."*

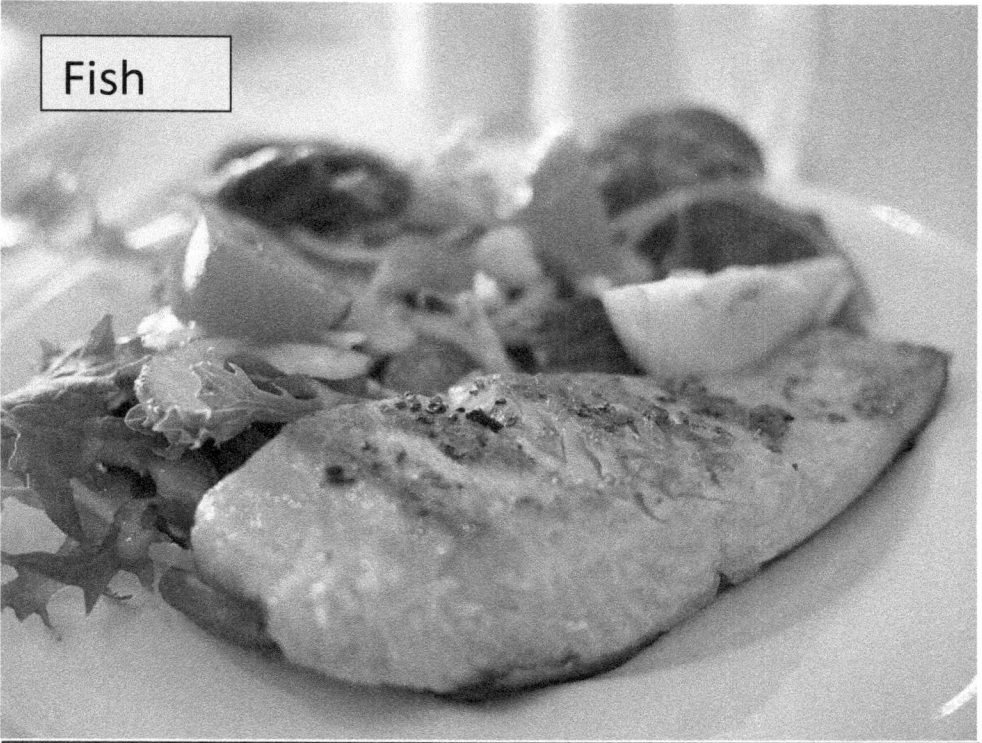

Fish

FISH

A 2012 study from *BMC Research Notes* compared the cardiovascular response in subjects consuming less than 70g of fish 2X per week to subjects consuming roughly 70g of fish 4X per week. While performing the stressful task of counting backward from 5000 by 13, the subjects consuming the fish 4X per week had lower blood pressure and heart rates during the stressful event (46).

Garlic

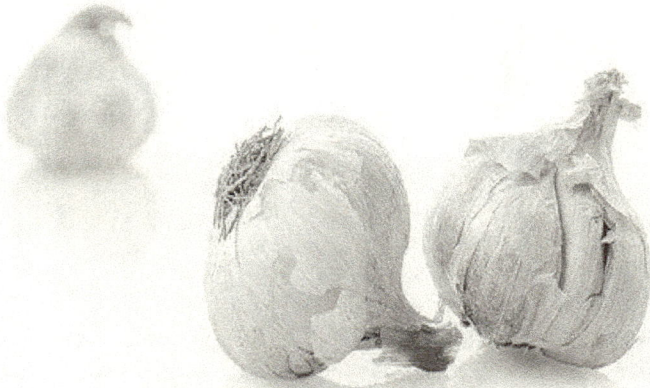

GARLIC

Garlic is loaded with antioxidants and contains Allicin which has been shown to fend off heart disease, cancer, and even common colds. A 2001 study from *The Journal of Nutrition* looked at the hormonal effects of supplementing with garlic while on a high protein diet. The researchers found that garlic may positively impact the anabolic hormonal effect of high protein diets by increasing testosterone and decreasing cortisol (54).

Green Tea

Hintzpeter J, Stapelfeld C, Loerz C, Martin H, Maser E. Green tea and one of its constituents, Epigallocatechine-3-gallate, are potent inhibitors of human 11B-hydroxysteroid dehydrogenase type 1. PLoS One. 9(1): e84468. 2014.

Enzyme 11-beta-HSD-1 converts inactive cortisone into active cortisol in the body. If interrupt 11-beta-HSD-1 in lab animals, they lose abdominal fat

Enzyme 11-beta-HSD-2, converts cortisol back into cortisone.

exposed liver cells to green, black and white tea then injected cortisone to the liver cells and measured cortisol levels. All three teas inhibited cortisol, but green tea had most significant impact.

Compounds epigallocatechin gallate (EGCG) and gallocatechin (GC) were found to be the cortisol inhibitors. "EGCG takes over the spot in the enzyme that is meant for cortisone, interrupting the conversion of cortisone into cortisol."

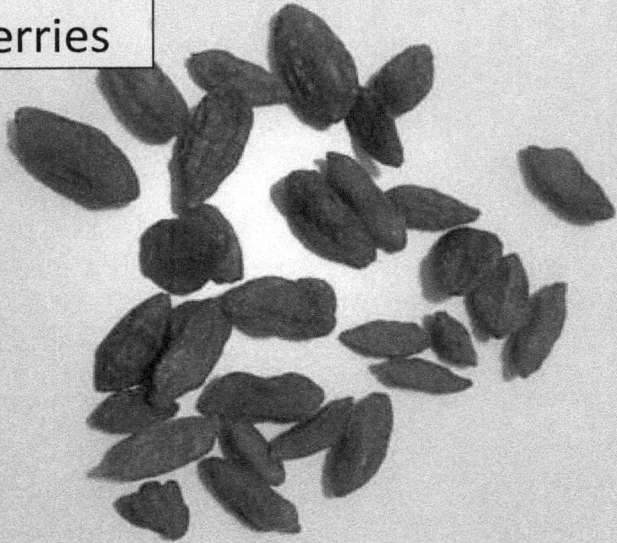

Goji Berries

<u>GOJI BERRIES</u>

A 2012 study from *PLoS One* gave rats either normal diet or polysaccharides from Goji berries for 3 weeks. After 3 weeks, the researchers then put the male rats into a cage with a female rat. The researchers found that the rats given the goji berries had much higher libido than those on the normal diets. In the second part of the study the rats were injected with cortisone. The cortisone had little to no effect on the goji berry rats as their testosterone was unaffected by the cortisone (41).

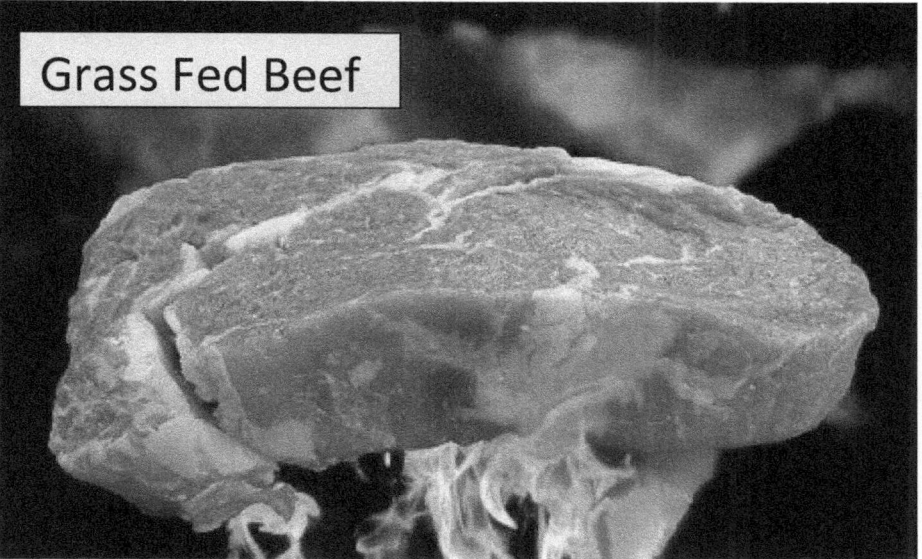
Grass Fed Beef

GRASS FED BEEF

- ➢ Grass fed only must eat grass 30% of the year. Green fed eat grass, herbs, legumes and other greens 100% of the year.
- ➢ More antioxidants
- ➢ Vitamin C, E, and beta carotene
- ➢ Does not have added hormones, antibiotics, or other drugs
- ➢ Two to four times healthier Omega 3 fatty acids
- ➢ Zinc, iron, and b vitamins that can help stabilize mood
- ➢ one of the most complete dietary sources of protein with the amino acid profile being almost identical to human muscle

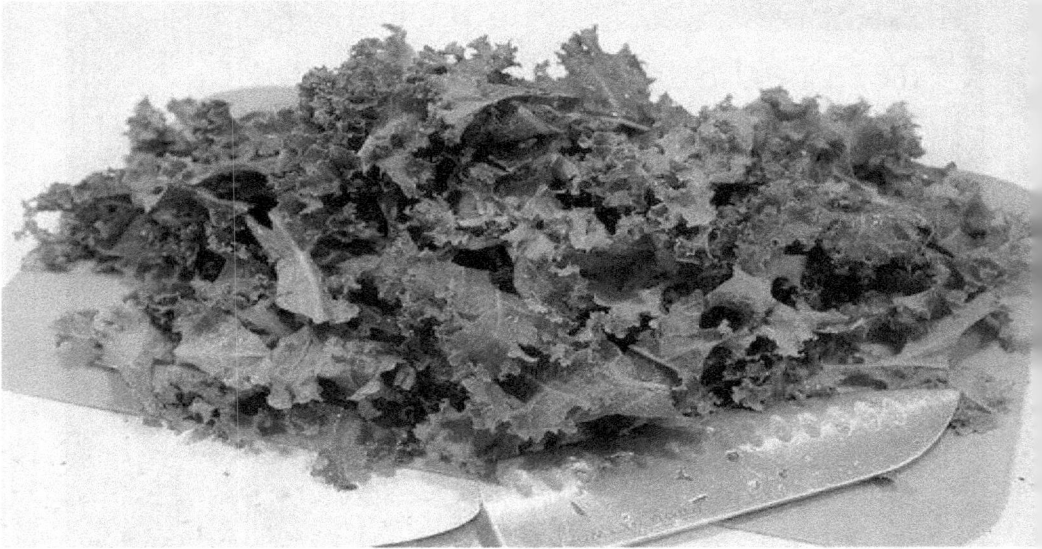

KALE

- Contains 206% daily requirement for vitamin A
- 135% vitamin C
- 684% vitamin K
- High in calcium, Magnesium Vitamin B 6, Lutein, and beta Carotene.

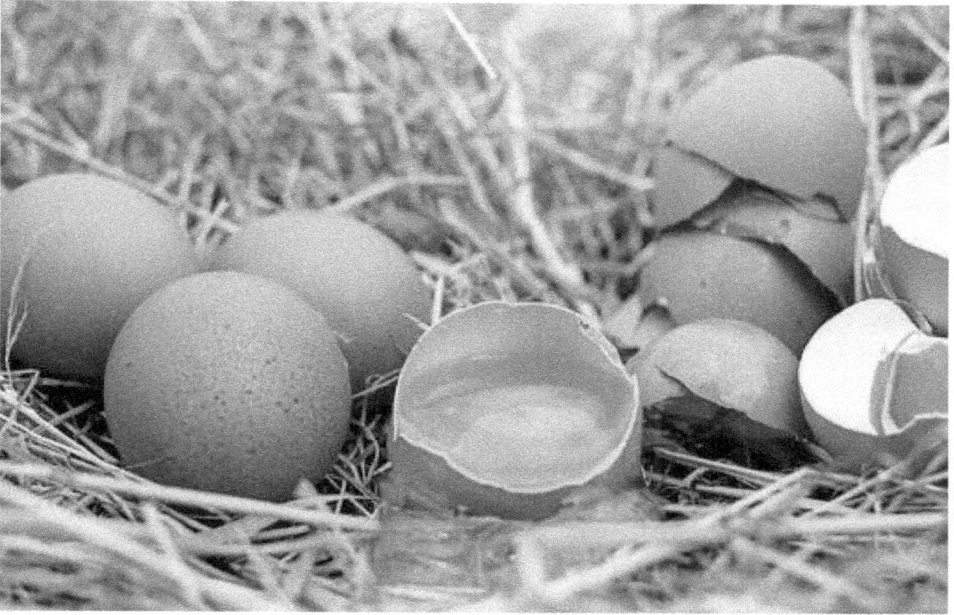

	Vitamin A (IU)	Vitamin E (mg)	Beta Carotene (mcg)	Omega-3s (g)	Cholesterol (mg)
Eggs from Confined Birds	487	0.97	10	0.22	423
Free Range Eggs	**791.86**	**3.73**	**79.03**	**0.66**	277

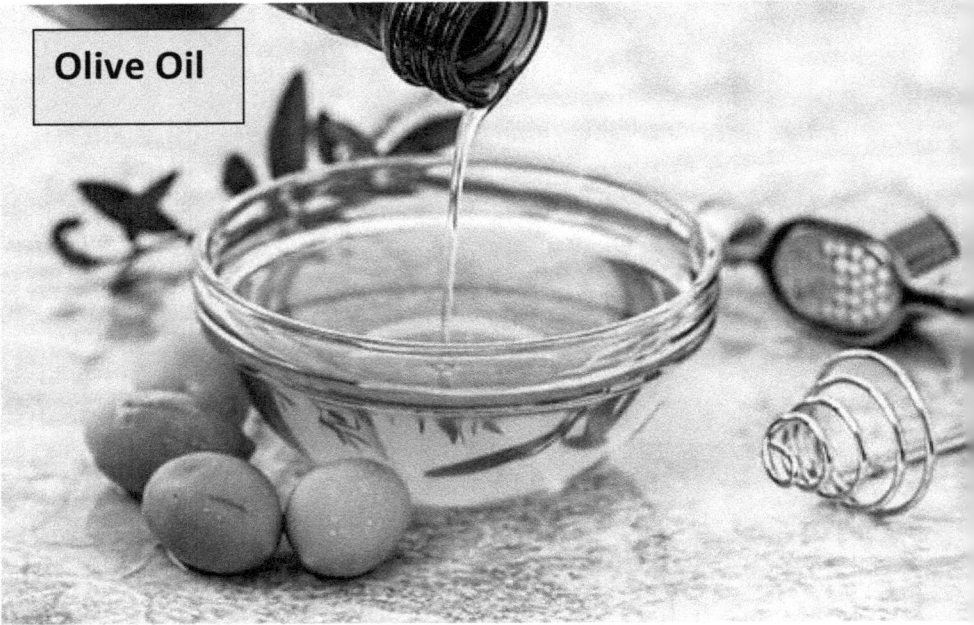

Olive Oil

OLIVE OIL

A 2013 study from the *Journal of Nutritional Biochemistry* looked at the effects a compound of olive oil, oleuropein, had on testosterone and cortisol levels. The researchers found that not only did the oleuropein increase testosterone and decrease cortisol levels, but it also helped the body absorb and retain proteins better, similar to the effects of garlic (55).

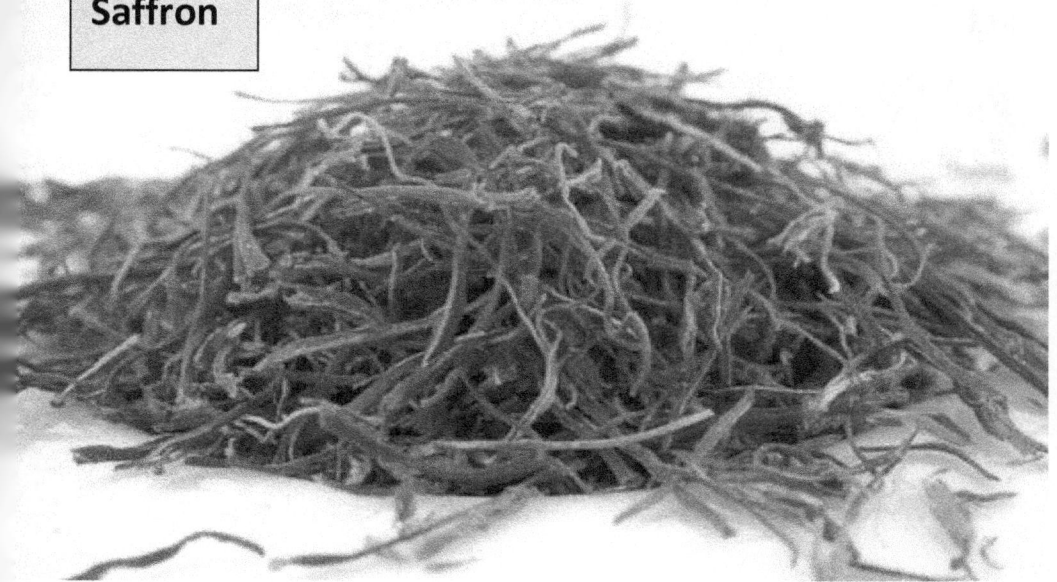

Saffron

Saffron

A 2011 study from *Phytomedicine* looked at the psychological and neuroendocrinological effects of aromatherapy with saffron. The researchers found that as little as 20 minutes of saffron aromatherapy decreased cortisol and anxiety symptoms in healthy female subjects (28).

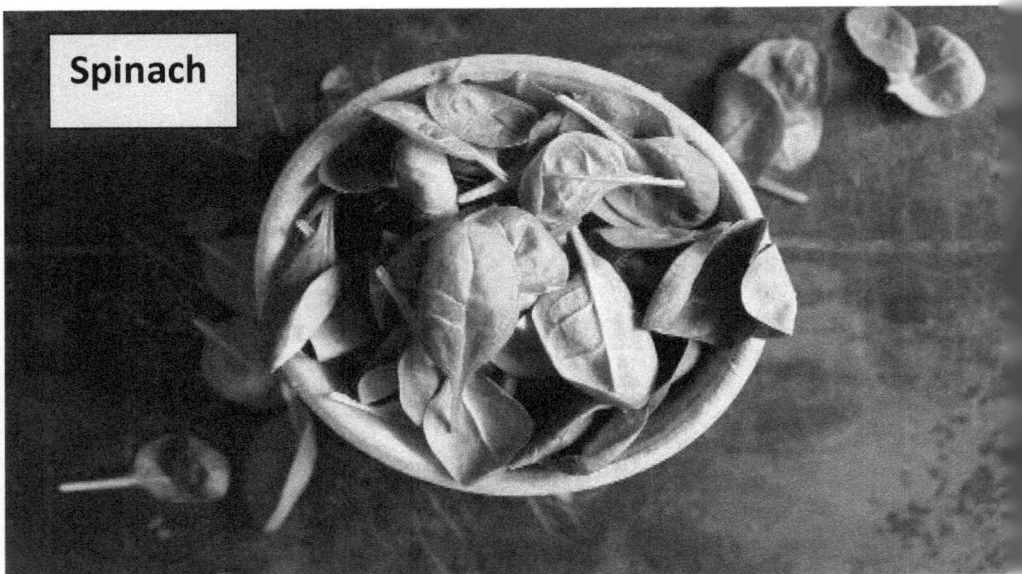
Spinach

Spinach

- ➤ High in vitamin C
- ➤ High in fiber and magnesium
- ➤ Great source of iron
- ➤ Source of folate
- ➤ Source of potassium
- ➤ Source of calcium

Sardines

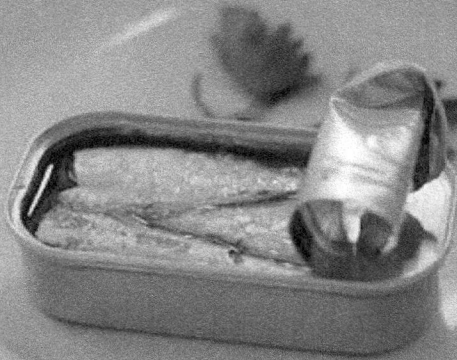

Sardines

- 36.7g protein
- 17.1g fat
- 2205mg omega-3 fatty acids (61%)
- 101% vitamin D
- 15% vitamin E
- 39% Niacin
- 222% B12
- 57% calcium (569mg)
- 73% Phosphorus (730mg)
- 112% Selenium (78.5mcg)
- 24% Iron (4.4mg)
- 15% Magnesium (58.1mg)
- 17% Potassium (592mg)
- 31% Sodium (752mg)
- 13% Zinc (2.0mg)
- 14% Copper (.3mg)

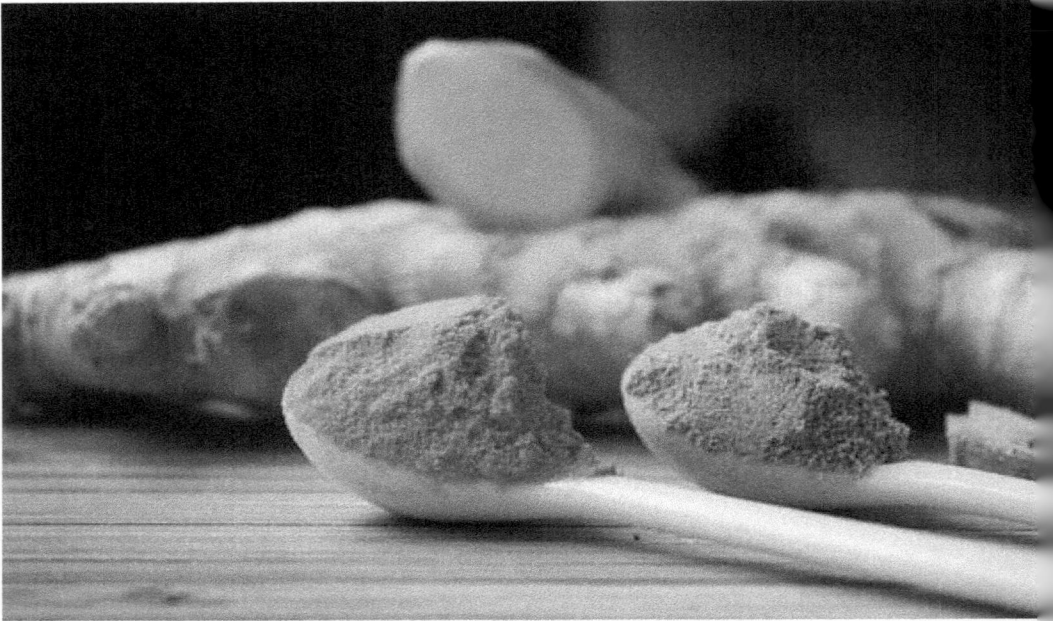

Turmeric

> ➤ Found in curcumin.
> ➤ 4th highest antioxidant rich herb.
> ➤ Great for fighting inflammation, improving blood flow, lowering stress, improving brain function/focus.

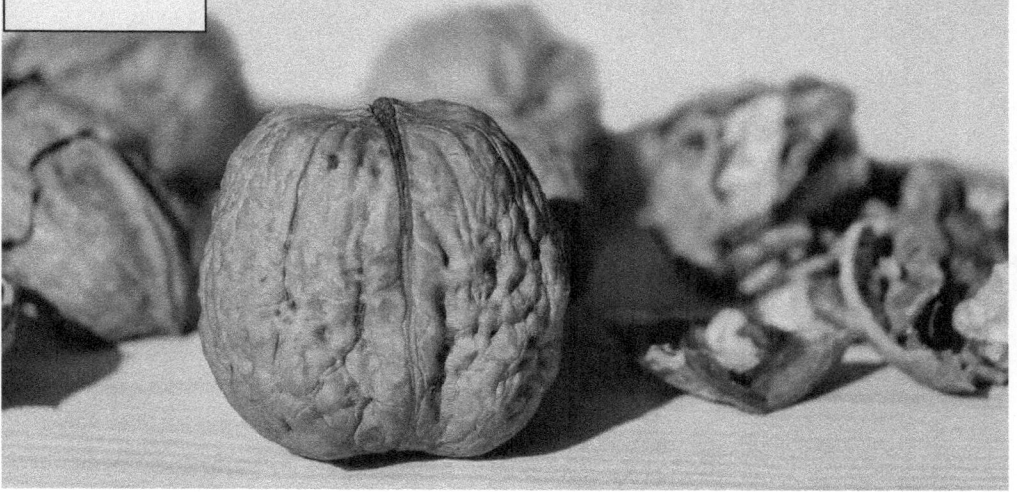

Walnuts

Walnuts

Walnuts are the only nuts that are high in the omega 3 fatty acid alpha linolenic acid. They are also a source of phosphorus, copper, manganese, vitamin E, B6, and B9. They also contain ellagic acid, catechins, and phytic acid. Walnuts even contain melatonin. 2014 study looked at the effects high consumption of fatty acids had on stress response. There were four separate dietary intervention groups: walnuts, chia seed, peanuts, and regular feed. The researchers found that the walnut and chia seed groups produced significantly less cortisol than the control and peanut groups (52).

ASSORTED ANTI-STRESS STRATEGIES

Balneo/Cold Water Therapy

From the Latin term *balneum*, or bath, balneotherapy has been used for centuries traced as far back as the Romans use of mineral springs throughout Europe. A 2006 study from *Biomedical Research* investigating the effect spa bathing had on salivary stress markers found that the Romans were indeed on to something, as the spa bathing decreased cortisol levels (78).

A study from 2010 in *Complementary Therapies in Medicine* compared which was better for treating generalized anxiety disorder: balneotherapy vs Paxil. You guessed it. The researchers found that the water baths were significantly more effective at improving the symptoms of generalized anxiety disorder than the common prescription medicine Paxil (19).

What about the cold water? The receptors in the body that respond to the cold have a much greater density, nearly 3X more, than the warm receptors. When stimulated, these cold receptors can have a significant effect, increasing blood flow to the brain and away from the extremities, stimulating the release of norepinephrine as well as several neurotransmitters. A 2008 study from *Medical Hypotheses* put this to the test as found that cold showers could improve depression symptoms (69).

Laugh/Smile

A 1989 study from the *American Journal of Medical Science* measured the endocrine response of five healthy male subjects during a sixty-minute comedy video and compared it to the response of five healthy males who did not watch the video. The group that watched the funny video had lower cortisol and epinephrine, leading the researchers to conclude the mirthful laughter was the cause (8).

Grin and Bear It. That was the title of a 2012 study from *Psychological Science* in which the researchers had the subjects perform stressful tasks while chopsticks were held in their mouths to form either a standard smile, a Duchenne smile, or a neutral facial expression. The researchers then asked half of the groups with the chopstick smiles to also voluntarily contract their smile muscles. The researchers found that all of the smiling groups, both voluntary and "chopstick" (involuntary) had lower heart rates in response to the stresses. The researchers concluded "there are both

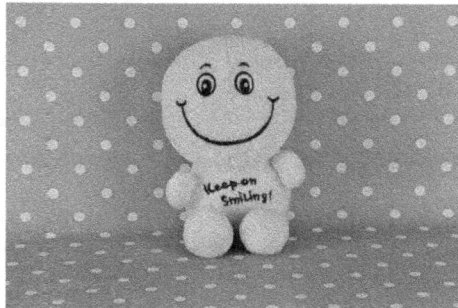

physiological and psychological benefits from maintaining positive facial expressions during stress (39)." *Hmmm, wonder if that explains the ever-present "smile" whenever left leaning politicians and pundits are interviewed on Fox News?*

Massage Therapy

Who doesn't love a good massage? Well did you know that a 2005 study from *The International Journal of Neuroscience* looked at the effects massage therapy had on cortisol and neurotransmitters. (Student at the campus center sign up bulletin*: "Hmmm, which study to I want to sign up for, the sprinting on the treadmill while wearing "Bane" mask from Dark Knight Rises, jumping into cold water wearing tri-colored speedo to measure blood flow distribution and reactivity, or the 60 - minute massage therapy?)* Anyway, the researchers found that massage treatments both increased serotonin levels and decreased cortisol levels (25).

Footbaths

Thomas Jefferson was apparently way ahead of his time. Per a 2008 study from *Complementary Therapies in Clinical Practice* footbaths can decrease stress and anxiety symptoms by relaxing the nervous system and decreasing stress hormones (84). In Chinese Medicine, it is believed that we draw energy from the earth and our feet are seen as our connection to the earth.

Dancing

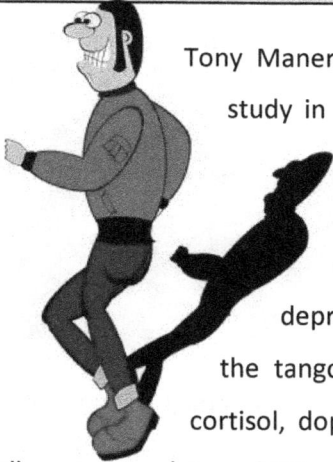

Who wins in a dance off Tony Manero or Napolean Dynamite? A 2009 study in *Music and Medicine* looked at the hormonal responses from 12 weeks of dancing in high school aged subjects suffering from depression. After 12 weeks of "dancing the tango" serotonin levels were up while cortisol, dopamine, and depression symptoms all dropped (61).

Chewing gum

A 2009 study from *Physiology and Behavior* found that during stressful times, chewing gum lowered cortisol and associated stress levels (33).

Chopping Wood

Did you know that an hour of hard manual labor can increase testosterone levels by almost 50%?

In a three month 2013 study from *Evolution and Human Behavior*, researchers tested the testosterone levels of horticultural tribesman in Bolivia before and after an hour of intense wood chopping. The researchers found that testosterone levels had increased an average of 48.6% after an hour of chopping wood. They concluded "when engaged in heavy physical activity, testosterone increases, allowing for the rapid muscular performance enhancement (80).

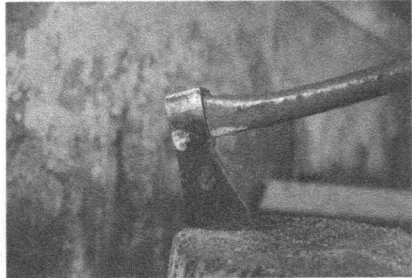

Meditate

According to a 1997 study from *Psychoneuroendocrinology,* four months of Transcendental Meditation elevated growth hormone levels while decreasing cortisol levels (45).

Gratitude Log

After only three weeks of keeping a grateful log subjects not only slept better, but they also slept longer. A 2003 study from the *Journal of Personality and Social Psychology* looked at these effects and concluded that *"a conscious focus on blessings may have emotional and interpersonal benefits (21)."*

A separate study, this one from 2011, found that as little as 15 minutes of writing in a gratitude log before going to bed led to better sleep and less worry in students (18).

Progressive Muscle Relaxation

Contracting a specific muscle group for seven seconds then completely relaxing those muscles for thirty seconds while focusing completely on the task at hand, can significantly lower cortisol levels. A 2002 study from *Biological Psychology* had subjects go through fifteen minutes of progressive muscle relaxation in the following order:

1. Upper right arm
2. Left lower arm
3. Left upper arm
4. Forehead
5. Muscles around the nose

6. Jaw muscles
7. Neck
8. Chest
9. Shoulders
10. Upper back
11. Stomach
12. Right leg
13. Left leg

The researchers found that this simple 15-minute routine dramatically cut cortisol levels (58).

Improving Posture

As we saw previously, holding a one minute "power pose" can increase testosterone while decreasing cortisol (10). The study reveals that by *"simply changing physical posture, an individual prepares his or her mental and physiological systems to endure difficult and stressful situations (10)."*

A 1998 study from *Behavioral and Brain Sciences* found that "expansive, open postures project high power, whereas contractive, closed postures project low power (49)." It has been shown that hunched over versus upright postures can lead feelings of depression (64).

Along with emphasizing structural balance in a weight training programme, excellent programs for postural correction include *Egoscue* and *Posturology*.

Increase Quality Fats

A 2014 study found that increasing poly unsaturated fatty acids, in the form of either chia seeds or walnuts, improved stress response and reactivity by decreasing cortisol levels (52).

Workout/Exercise

Paying credence to the belief that the human body is made for motion, a 2015 study from *Psychoneuroendocrinology* found that ""*physical exercise activated the hippocampus, inactivated the prefrontal cortex, and reduced the cortisol response to an emotional task. Physical exercise might thus enhance resilience by regulating the hypothalamic-pituitary-adrenal axis to buffer the effect of daily tress. Physical exercise may therefore prevent depression by promoting resilience (86).*"

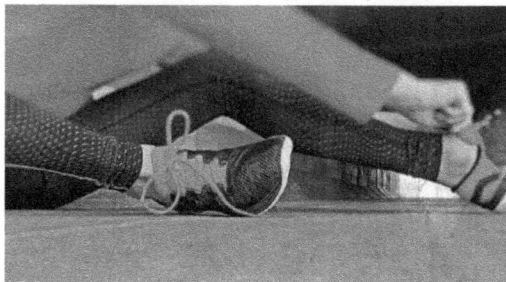

Exercise can increase cognitive function and stress tolerance while improving mood through the effects of the hormones and neurohormones released as a result of a good workout.

Childs et al found that *"regular exercisers are more resistant to the emotional effects of acute stress, which in turn, may protect them against diseases related to chronic stress burden (13)."*

BDNF

Brain-Derived Neurotrophic Factor. BNDF is a neurotrophic protein that plays an important role in neuroplasticity, cognitive function, nervous system functioning, neuronal production, memory, and more.

Physical activity stimulates the release of BDNF, as does cold water immersion, sun exposure, certain foods including cocoa, fish oil, and blueberries, as well as a few supplements including magnesium, curcumin, L-theanine, Ginseng, Bacopa, Rhodiola, and EGCG.

Learning has also been shown to increase BDNF which in turn enhances more learning (79). A 1999 study from *Proceedings of the National Academy of Sciences* found that running, which stimulates BDNF, enhances neurogenesis and learning (82).

For more on BDNF, I recommend reading the book *SPARK* by Dr. John J. Ratey.

Strength Training

Strength training can dramatically improve one's hormonal profile. A 2007 study from the *European Journal of Applied Physiology* had 20 beginner weight training subjects undergo 4 weeks of strength training three times per week. After 4 weeks, the researchers found decreased cortisol and nearly 40% increases in resting testosterone (3). Other studies have had similar findings (7).

Manage Pain

PROTEOLYTIC ENZYMES
BROMELAIN (FROM PINEAPPLE)
PAPAIN (FROM PAPAYA)
TRYPSIN AND CHYMOTRYPSIN (ALSO FROM PINEAPPLE), **SERRATIA PEPTIDASE** (FROM SILK WORM)

Miller P, Bailey S, Barnes M, Derr S, Hall E. **The effects of protease supplementation on skeletal muscle function and DOMS following downhill running.** *J Sports Sci.* 22*4); Pp 365-372. 2004.

- seven enzyme mixture 4 times per day between 24 and 96 hours after their downhill running bout, or a placebo. The enzyme group "demonstrated superior recovery of contractile function and diminished effect of DOMS". The researchers concluded that "protease supplementation may also facilitate muscle healing and allow for faster restoration of contractile function after intense exercise".

Beck T, Housh T, Johnson G, Schmidt R< Housh D, Coburn J, Malek M, Mielke M. **Effects of a protease supplement on eccentric exercise induced markers of delayed onset muscle soreness and muscle damage.** *Journal of Strength and Conditioning Research.* 21(3); Pp 661-667. 2007.

- double-blind, placebo controlled method of scientific research. The researchers found a much more rapid recovery from the workout as well as a decreased loss of strength immediately after the workout.

Donath F, Mai I, Maurer A, Brockmoller J, Kuhn C, Friedrich G, Roots I. **Dose-related bioavailability of bromelain and trypsin after repeated oral administration.** *Am S Clin Pharmacol and Therap.* 61; Pp 157. 1997

- proteolytic enzymes effectively absorbed large protein molecules, theorizing this to be part of the effectiveness of these enzymes in fighting inflammation and bruising.

Boswellic acids were found to decrease the pain and inflammation associated with arthritis (2). A double-blind placebo controlled study found significant improvements in asthma symptoms after just six weeks of Boswellia gum treatment (32).

Ginger extract has also been shown to be effective in managing pain. After six weeks of receiving ginger extract, 261 patients with osteoarthritis saw significant improvement in their knee pain versus those subjects taking a placebo (1).

Capsaicin has also been seen as a novel treatment for osteoarthritis knee pain (27). as it *"targets specific pathways involved inflammation through a multitude of actions (66)."*

Passionflower has also shown promise in pain management. Per a 2008 study on Passionflower, the authors express *"with this radical, scavenging ability, a decrease in inflammation can be a desirable side effect (47)."*

Hydrate

Drinking water during 90 minute workouts led to less cortisol being produced and had a positive effect on fat burning (5). Speaking of hydrating during a workout and fat burning, a 2003 study from the *European Journal of Clinical Nutrition* found that when muscle cells were hydrated they were more efficient in protecting proteins from breaking down. The researchers also found that when fat cells were hydrated they were more efficient at releasing fats (40).

Morning Light Exposure

Exposure to artificial morning light can positively impact cortisol levels. A 2013 study from *Chronobiology International* found artificial morning light to have a positive effect on mood, well-being, cognitive performance, melatonin levels and cortisol (29).

Supplement with Fish Oil

According to a 2013 randomized, placebo-controlled study from *Molecular Nutrition and Food Research* supplementing with fish oil can decrease ratings of perceived stress and lower cortisol levels (6).

ANTIOXIDANTS

Vitamin E	Vegetables, Fish Oils, some fruits, seeds and nuts, and whole grains	Fat soluble vitamin, has been found to be one of the most abundant and potent scavengers of free radicals. Plays role in decreased risk of degenerative diseases and cancer. Can be recycled by Vitamin C and Alpha Lipoic Acid. Recommended to take vitamin E that contains all members of vitamin E family, 4 tocopherols and 4 tocotrienols.
Vitamin C	Broccoli, spinach, cabbage, kale, green peppers, citrus fruits, and citrus juices.	Can regenerate vitamin E to improve overall antioxidant capacity. May help to reduce inflammation and improve immune health. Deficiencies have been shown to be a risk factor in CVD and oxidative stress.
Vitamin A	Cod liver oil, broccoli, carrots, eggs, kale, animal liver, and sweet potatoes	Known for eye health, vitamin A is also very important for blood cell development and immune health. Healthy skin is also associated with Vitamin A levels.
CoQ10	Animal liver, cold water fish, walnuts,	Can also recycle vitamin E. Known for its role in cardiovascular health through its effects on energy production and

	grapeseed and olive oils	mitochondrial health. Studies have shown CoQ10 plays a role in neurodegenerative diseases, cancer and diabetes. It has also been shown to be a treatment for migraine headaches.
EGCG	Green Tea, white tea, and black tea.	Shown to be potent antioxidant in combatting neurodegenerative diseases and inflammation. Also, it has been shown to stimulate testosterone production and be cancer protectant.
Pycnogenol	French maritime pine bark	This potent antioxidant scavenger has been shown to play a role in decreasing inflammation. Has been shown to slightly increase salivary testosterone and play a role in combatting erectile dysfunction.
Alpha Lipoic Acid	Animal kidney, heart, and liver, spinach, broccoli, and Brussel sprouts.	Has been shown to play a role in generation of the body's most powerful endogenous antioxidant, glutathione. Studies have shown can regenerate both vitamin E and C, making this a potent tool in combatting inflammation, oxidative stress, and improving mitochondrial health. Recommended to purchase R-stabilized form of ALA.

Resveratrol	Red wine, white wine, blueberries, red grapes	Has been shown to have positive effects on neurodegeneration, inflammation, and cardiovascular health. It has also been shown to have anti-estrogenic and anti-carcinogenic properties.
EGCG	Green and White Teas	Has been shown to have anti-carcinogenic and anti-inflammatory properties and can potentially increase the activity of endogenous antioxidants.
Chlorogenic Acids	Coffee, prunes, peaches	Anti-inflammatory and cardiovascular health benefits.
Flavanols: procyanidins epicatechins and catechins	Dark Chocolate, Berries, Kale, Broccoli	Cardiovascular health, anti-carcinogenic, and anti-inflammatory benefits.
Anthocyanins	Cherries, Prunes, Acai Berry	Anti-degenerative, cardiovascular and anti-inflammatory health benefits.
Zinc	Oysters, Polyrachis Ant, Beef, Spinach, Wheat Germ, cashews,	Research has shown zinc to be a potent antioxidant associated with immune function and health.

	Dark Chocolate	
Manganese	Mussels, Nuts, Seeds, Spinach, Kale	Major building block for one of body's most potent endogenous antioxidant, superoxide dismutase.
Carotenoids: Lycopene, beta-carotene, Lutein, Astaxanthin	Tomatoes, Peppers, Guavas, Grapefruit, Salmon, Winter Squash, Okra, Kale, Beef	Anti-inflammatory, anti-carcinogenic effects and cardiovascular health benefits.
Capsaicin	Chili Peppers	Regulation of blood sugar, anti-arthritic, anti-inflammatory, and potential anti-carcinogenic properties

VITAMINS, MINERALS, AND SUPPLEMENTS

Vitamin C

A study from 2008 looked at the effects 1000 mg of vitamin C had on post exercise inflammation, muscle damage, and cortisol levels. Between 2 and 24 hours after a thirty-minute workout at 75% Vo2 Max, cortisol levels were significantly lower while inflammation was lower at the 24-hr. post mark (51).

Another study set out to test how subjects would respond to psychological stress after being exposed to two stressful events. For fourteen days' subjects received either placebo or 1000mg of ascorbic three times per day. After fourteen days, the group receiving ascorbic acid had lower blood pressure, lower cortisol, and less perceived stress in response to the stressful events (9).

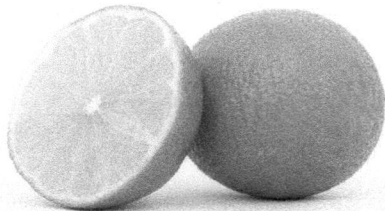

A third study, this one from 2001, had ultramarathoners supplement with a placebo or 1000mg vitamin C per day, with blood work being taken 16 hours before, 30 min, 24 hour, and 48 hours after the race. The vitamin C group had significantly lower cortisol levels than the placebo group post-race (59).

Vitamin D

By 2020 will vitamin D still be referred to as a vitamin, or a hormone, or something in between? A 2012 study titled Vitamin D in acute stress and critical illness found that *"variations in patient responses to acute stress and critical illness may depend on the degree of vitamin D insufficiency and extent of tissue requirement (60)."*

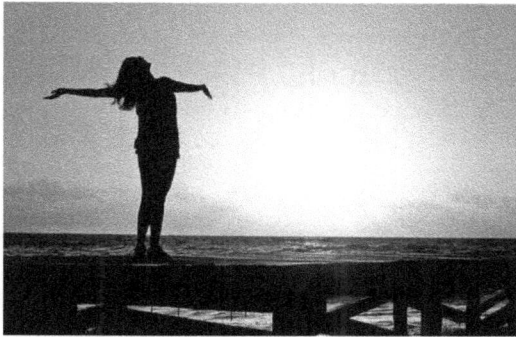

Vitamin D has been linked to everything from cardiovascular events and mortality, to diabetes, obesity and several types of cancer (48). There are three ways to maintain vitamin D status, through sunshine, diet, or pharmaceutical/supplement (48).

CoQ10

CoQ10 is a potent antioxidant that can regenerate other antioxidants including Vitamin E and C. Just 200mg was shown to lower systolic blood pressure by 11mmHG and diastolic by 7mmHG in just three weeks (85).

Magnesium

Did you know that magnesium is a cofactor in over 300 enzymatic reactions? Magnesium plays a role testosterone bioavailability and production, calcium absorption (23), stress reduction (53), and cortisol production/regulation (62).

Amino Acids

In 2010 researchers found that consuming 3g of branch chained amino acids for three weeks lowered cortisol levels while raising testosterone levels 12 hours post workout (68).

NAC/Selenium

N-acetyl-cysteine is a modified version of the amino acid cysteine that plays a role in glutathione replenishment and antioxidant defenses. Selenium is a cofactor in the production of glutathione. When taken together at 200 mcg of selenium and 600 mg of NAC, for 26-weeks subjects saw significant increases in testosterone levels (65).

Grape Seed Extract

Grape seeds are loaded with antioxidants in the form of ogilomeric proanthocyanidin complexes, or OPC for short. Grape seed extract has been shown to lower cortisol while elevating testosterone through its suppressive effects on aromatase.

Phosphatidylserine

Phosphatidylserine is a phospholipid that has been shown to have a positive effect on cortisol. A 2008 study had subjects take 600 mg of phosphatidylserine for ten days and found both an increase in testosterone and decrease in cortisol after moderate intensity exercise (73).

L-Theanine

L-Theanine, an amino acid found in green tea, has been shown in research to stimulate alpha wave release. These alpha waves help the brain to both concentrate and relax (71). A 2007 study from *Biological Psychology* found that just 200mg of theanine could decrease heart rate and feelings of anxiety during stressful situations (38).

L-Lysine/L- Arginine

L-Lysine is an essential amino acid while L-Arginine is essential/semi-essential. A 2007 study had subjects take 2.3 grams of L-Lysine and L-Arginine for 7 seven days and found a significant drop in morning cortisol after only a week (70).

Holy Basil

Holy Basil (Tulsi) has been referred to as an *"herb for all reasons"*, as it has been used for everything from rebalancing hormones and normalizing neurotransmitters to combatting metabolic, physical, and mental stress. A 2014 study aptly titled Tulsi-Ocimum sanctum: A herb for all reasons shows that holy basil can lead to a significant drop in fasting glucose, cholesterol levels, and stress. The study also points out that *"The phytochemicals in tulsi prevent chemical induced skin, liver, oral and lung cancers because they increase antioxidant activity, alter healthy gene expressions, induce cancer cell death, prevent blood vessel growth contributing to cell grown and stop metastasis (15)."*

Rhodiola Rosea

100mg of the adaptogen herb Rhodiola for twenty days has been shown decrease stress levels and improve feelings of well-being (72). A separate study, this one from 2012 in Phytotherapy Research found that 400mg of Rhodiola broken down into two 200mg dosages for 4 weeks improved well-being while reducing stress levels (20).

Ginkgo Biloba

A 2002 study looked at the effect ginkgo had on blood pressure and cortisol under stressful situations. Researchers had subjects take 120 mg of ginkgo or a placebo thirty minutes before mentally and physically stressful situation. The researchers found the ginkgo not only had a positive impact on blood pressure, but also inhibited the production of cortisol (36).

Passionflower and Lemon Balm

Through its effects on the inhibitory neurotransmitter GABA, 300 mg of lemon balm for just 15 days has been shown to improve sleep quality while decreasing anxiety ratings (11). A separate study from the International Journal of Clinical and Experimental Medicine had similar findings (24).

Magnolia Bark

Through its actions on GABA, just 500 mg of Magnolia bark per day for 4 weeks, resulted in a significant inhibition of cortisol alongside improvement in mood stability during stressful situations (76).

Quercetin

Quercitin is a flavanol found in some vegetables, sweet potatoes, capers, cilantro, onions, and tea. Researchers found Quercetin to have an inhibitory effect on cortisol production when taken before stressful events (37).

Ashwagandha

Ashwagandha is a popular herb in Ayurvedic medicine. A study from 2009 in *PLoS One* found that 600 mg of Ashwagandha a day for eight weeks saw a significant drop in anxiety (16), while a 2000 study saw a similar result with just six weeks of 500 mg Ashwagandha per day (4). A randomized, double-blind, placebo-controlled study from 2012 saw nearly a 30% drop in cortisol with 300 mg Ashwagandha for roughly eight weeks (12).

Tongkat Ali

Otherwise known as *Eurycoma longifolia*, Tongkat Ali has been shown in research to increase both free and total testosterone in as little as five weeks. Dosage was 400mg per day (34). A separate study from *The Journal of International Society of*

Sports Nutrition found both an inhibition of cortisol and a rise in testosterone levels with 200mg of Tongkat Ali for four weeks (77).

Panax Ginseng

A 2011 study from the *Journal of Ginseng Research* found that red ginseng could decrease stress and cortisol levels while improving mood and well-being (14).

Horny Goat Weed

The flavanol Icariin, found in horny goat weed, was investigated for its purported effects on the hypothalamic-pituitary-adrenal axis under times of stress. In 2006 researchers found that Icariin significantly inhibited cortisol production (57).

Lavender

Lavender has been found to decrease cortisol levels (26). A 2010 study found that 80 mg of Lavender per day for six weeks improved symptoms of generalized anxiety disorder (83). A 2012 study found Lavender to decrease blood pressure (67), while a study from 2005 found it to improve quality of sleep while decreasing insomnia symptoms (44).

Melatonin

A double bind study from 2009 in Psychopharmacology found that 3 mg of melatonin taken prior, improved cognition and memory during a stressful event (63).

CHAPTER 4: SIMPLE CHANGES

START THE DAY OFF WITH A WIN

1. Make your bed as soon as you wake up.

The importance of this simple task was explained by Navy SEAL and Naval Admiral Wiliam McRaven at his University of Texas, Austin graduation commencement speech (Mudallal 2015) *"If you make your bed every morning, you will have accomplished the first task of the day. It will give you a small sense of pride and it will encourage you to do another task and another and another. By the end of the day, that one task completed will have turned into many tasks completed. Making your bed will also reinforce the fact that little things in life matter. It helps with the clutter and visual appeal of your room. This is an obvious one, but way overlooked. Your room is your sanctuary, and a decluttered space is proved to reduce stress (7)".*

2. Drink 10- 16oz of water with lime Himalayan Sea Salt.

➢ Vitamin C is a potent antioxidant, essential in liver detoxification through it role in glutathione production, and has been shown in several studies to lower cortisol."

➢ Himalayan Salt contains roughly 84 trace minerals that can be used by the body for numerous chemical and enzymatic reactions.

➢ Salt has very strong anti-microbial properties

➢ Salt and lime can stimulate the body to become more alkaline after becoming more acidic during the night.

➢ Limes are god for the joints as they can help rid them of uric acid

➢ Can improve digestion by hydrating and clearing toxins, as well improve immune function

3. Workout

➢ Through its effects on BDNF
  - o exercise promotes a higher order of brain plasticity and learning ability (11)
  - o Physical activity was associated with lower risks of cognitive impairment, Alzheimer's, and dementia (6)
  - o Exercise enhances learning (12)

- o Exercise promotes brain vascularization (5)
- ➤ Through its effects on hormones
  - o Testosterone levels were nearly 40% higher, while cortisol levels were significantly lower after just 4 weeks of strength training *(2)"*

4. Eat a high-quality fat and protein breakfast

- ➤ High quality fat/low carb breakfast produced less cortisol, as diets high in poly unsaturated fats have been shown to play a positive role in modulating physiological and psychological stress responses (Nemeth et al 2014)
- ➤ Quality fats and proteins including pasteurized eggs, wild caught fish, grass fed beef, hormone and antibiotic free range chicken, avocados, nuts, and seeds stimulate dopamine and acetylcholine, the neurotransmitters associated with decision making, attention, reaction time, motivation, arousal, and cognitive/motor control.
- ➤ Examples include: baked avocado and eggs, organic bacon and free range eggs, salmon and walnuts, steak and almonds, chicken and avocado

5. End your shower with cold water

- ➤ Cold water has a stimulatory effect on both your neurotransmitter production and blood flow to the brain (10).

FOCUS ON AMBITIONS

Daily ambitions, weekly ambitions, monthly, etc. Working toward an ambition keeps us moving forward rather than looking back. Being productive builds confidence, which in turn alleviates stress.

1. Start with a clean space

> ➤ A study from 2010 in *Personality and Social Psychology Bulletin* found that *"wives who described their homes as being more stressful (that is, who talked more about clutter and unfinished projects) had marginally lower*

marital satisfaction. Wives who described their homes as more stressful also had flatter diurnal slopes of cortisol, an indicator of chronic stress that has been linked with adverse health outcomes. They also tended to show greater increases in depressed mood across the day, consistent with greater fatigue in the evening and a more difficult transition from work to home. In contrast, wives who described their homes as more restorative (that is, who talked more about their yards and outdoor home features, and who used more words connoting relaxation at home) had steeper diurnal cortisol slopes and showed decreased depressed mood across the day (9)."

2. Checklists

➤ Checklists can alleviate stress by allowing us to stay organized and not forget about things. A 2006 study titled *The Checklist – a tool for error management and performance improvement* found that creating and completing checklists significantly improved outcomes, decreased mistakes, and improved morale (4).

3. Deconstruct the stress

➤ In the "life" game of chess against stress, analyzing/deconstructing the moves made against you, placing a value on these moves, and determining the proper response/countermove can positively impact our ability to cope stressful situations. A Navy Special Warfare Combatant-craft Crewman friend of mine explains it simply as *"keeping your head over your feet at all times."* In other words, focusing on the task at hand, deconstructing the situation, and figuring out a solution.

END THE DAY ON A POSITIVE NOTE

Ending the day on a positive note can go a long way in ensuring good night's sleep. A few strategies to getting a better night's sleep include:

1. Magnesium before bed:

> Magnesium has been shown in research to decrease cortisol on alleviate stress symptoms and decrease cortisol. A 2012 study from the *Journal of Research in Medical Sciences* found that magresium can significantly improve measures of insomnia including sleep time, onset of sleep, and deep sleep [1]

2. 15-minute Progressive Muscle Relaxation

> Contracting a specific muscle group for seven seconds then completely relaxing those muscles for thirty seconds while focusing completely on the task at hand, can significantly lower cortisol levels (8).

3. Write down the things you are/were grateful for

> A 2011 study found that as little as 15 minutes of writing in a gratitude log before going to bed led to better sleep and less worry in students (3).

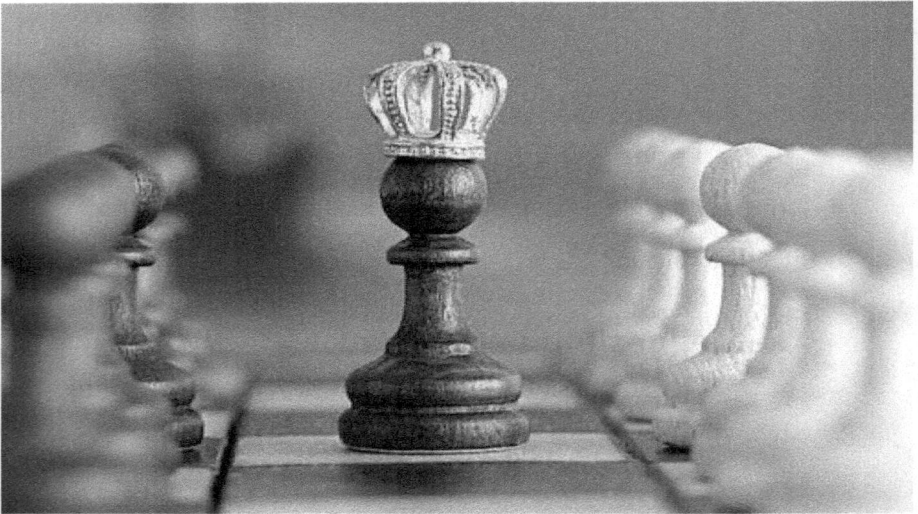

Chapter 1 References

1. Archer J. **Testosterone and human aggression: An evaluation of the challenge hypothesis.** *Neuroscience and Behavioral Reviews.* 30; Pp 319-345. 2006.

2. Badrick E, Bobak M, Britton A, Kirchbaum C, Marmot M, Kumari M. **The relationship between alcohol consumption and cortisol secretion in an aging cohort.** *J Clin Endocrinol Metab.* 93(3); Pp 750-757. 2008.

3. Bocarsly M, Powell E, Avena N, Hoebel B. **High fructose corn syrup causes characteristics of obesity in rats: increased body weight, body fat and triglyceride levels.** *Pharmacol Biochem Behav.* 97(1); Pp 101-106. 2010.

4. Blum C. **The relationship between the pelvis and stomatognathic system: A position statement.** *SOTO.* Pp 40-43. Oct 23-26, 2008.

5. Camfield D, Wetherell M, Scholey A, Cox K, Fogg E, White D, Sams J, Kras M, Stough C, Sali A, Pipingas A. **The effects of multivitamin supplementation on diurnal cortisol secretion and perceived stress.** *Nutrients.* 5(11); Pp 4429-4450. 2013.

6. Carney D, Cuddy A, Yap A. **Power Posing: Brief nonverbal displays affect neuroendocrine levels and risk tolerance.** *Psychological Science Online.* Pp 1-6. 2010.

7. Cohen R. Vasavada A, Wiest M, Schmitter-Edgecombe M. **Mobility and upright posture are associated with different aspects of cognition in older adults** *Frontiers in Aging Neuroscience.* 8(257); Pp 1-8. 2016.

8. Costa G, Pickup L, Di Martino V. **Commuting—a further stress factor for working people: evidence from the European Community. I. A review.** *International Archives of Occupational and Environmental Health.* 60(5); Pp 371-376. 1988.

9. Costa G, Pickup L, Di Martino V. **Commuting—a further stress factor for working people: evidence from the European Community. II. An empirical study.** *International Archives of Occupational and Environmental Health.* 60(5); Pp 377-385. 1988.

10. Delarue J, Matzinger O, Binnert C, Schneiter P, Chiolero R, Tappy L. **Fish oil prevents the adrenal activation elicited by mental stress in healthy men.** *Diabetes and Metabolism.* 29(3); Pp 289-295. 2003.

11. Diamanti-Kandarakis E, Bourguignon J, Guidice L, Hauser R, Prins G, Soto A, Zoeller T, Gore A. **Endocrine-disrupting chemicals: an endocrine society scientific statement.** *Endocrine Review.* 30(4); Pp 293-342. 2009

12. Diaz E, Ruiz F, Hoyos I, Zubero J, Gravina L, Gil J, Irazusta J, Gil S. **Cell damage, antioxidant status, and cortisol levels related to nutrition**

in ski mountaineering during a two-day race. *Journal of Sport Sciences and Medicine.* 9; Pp 338-346.

13. Dufault R, Leblanc B, Schnoll R, Cornett C, Schweitzer L, Wallinga D, Hightower J, Patrick L, Lukiw W. **Mercury from chlor-alkali plants: measured concentrations in food product sugar.** *Environmental Health.* 26(8); Pp 2. 2009.

14. Duong M, Cohen J, Convit A. **High cortisol levels are associated with low quality food choice in Type 2 Diabetes.** *Endocrine.* 41(1); Pp 76-81. 2012.

15. Epel E, McEwen B, Seeman T, Mathews K, Castellazzo G, Brownell K, Bell J, Ickovics J. **Stress and body shape: stress-induced cortisol secretion is consistently greater among women with central fat.** *Psychosomatic Medicine.* 62(5); Pp 623-632. 2000.

16. Epel E, Moyer A, Martin C, Macary S, Cummings N, Rodin J, Rebuffe-Scrive M. **Stress induced cortisol response and fat distribution in women.** *Obesity Research.* 2(3);Pp 255-262. 1994.

17. Epel E, Moyer A, Martin C, Macary S, Cummings N, Rodin J, Rebuffe-Scrive M. **Stress induced cortisol, mood, and fat distribution in men.** *Obesity Research.* 7(1); Pp 9-15. 1999.

18. Evans G, Wener R. **Rail commuting duration and passenger stress.** *J Autism Dev Disord.* 25(3); Pp 408-412. 2006.

19. Farhanghi M, Mahboob S, Ostadrahimi A. **Obesity induced magnesium deficiency can be treated by vitamin D supplementation.** *The Journal of the Pakistan Medical Association.* 59(4); Pp 258-261. 2009.

20. Fisher M, Ridelinger K, Gutenbrunner C, Bernateck M. **Influence of the tempomandibular joint on range of motion of the hip joint in patients with complex regional pain syndrome.** *J Manipulative Physicol Ther.* 32(5); Pp 364-371. 2009.

21. Grosso G, Galvano F, Marventano S, Malaguarnera M, Bucolo C, Drago F, Caraci F. **Omega-3 fatty acids and depression: scientific evidence and biological mechanisms.** *Oxid Med Cell Longev.* 313570. 2014.

22. Hall S, Aisbett B, Tait J, Turner A, Ferguson S, Main L. **The acute physiological stress response to an emergency alarm and mobilization during the day and at night.** *Noise Health.* 18(82); Pp 150-156. 2016.

23. Hofkosh-Hulbert E. **Connecting Tension in the hips and jaw.** www.cnmwellness.com. April 17, 2012.

24. Institute for Agriculture and Trade Policy. **Much High Fructose Corn Syrup Contaminated with Mercury, New Study Finds Brand-Name Food Products Also Discovered to Contain Mercury.** *Institute for Agriculture and Trade Policy Report.* January 26, 2009.

25. Irfan Y. **Associations among dehydration, testosterone and stress hormones in terms of body weight loss before competition.** *The American Journal of the Medical Sciences.* 350(2); Pp 103-108. 2015

26. Junta Takamatsu, Motoko Majima, Kyoko Miki, Kanji Kuma And Toshiji Mozai. **Serum Ferritin as a Marker of Thyroid Hormone Action on Peripheral Tissues.** *The Journal of Clinical Endocrinology & Metabolism* Vol. 61, No. 4 672-676, 1985.

27. Kajantie E, Phillips D. **The effects of sex and hormonal status on the physiological response to acute psychosocial stress.** *Psychoneuroendocrinology.* 31(2); Pp 151-178. 2006.

28. Kudieka B, Buske-Kirschbaum A, Hellhammer D, Kirschbaum C. **HPA axis responses to laboratory psychosocial stress in healthy elderly adults, younger adults, and children: impact of age and gender.** *Pscyhoneuroendocrinology.* 29(1); Pp 83-98. 2004.

29. Kraemer W, Solomon-Hill G, et al. **The effects of soy and whey protein supplementation on acute hormonal responses to resistance exercise in men.** *The Journal of the American College of Nutrition.* 32(1); Pp 66-74. 2013.

30. Le M, Frye R, Rivard C, Cheng J, McFann K, Segal M, Johnson R, Johnson J. **Effects of high-fructose corn syrup and sucrose on the pharmacokinetics of fructose and acute metabolic and hemodynamic responses in health subjects.** *Metabolism.* 61(5)); Pp 641-651. 2012.

31. Lee P. **Vitamin D metabolism and deficiency in critical illness.** *Best Pract Res Clin Endocrinol Metab.* 25; Pp 769-781. 2011.

32. Leproult R, Copinschi G, Buxton O, Van Cauter E. **Sleep loss results in an elevation of cortisol levels the next evening.** *Sleep.* 20(10); Pp 865-870. 1997.

33. Liu H, Huang D, Mcarthur D, Boros L, Nissen N, Heaney A. **Fructose induces transketolase flux to promote pancreatic cancer growth.** *Cancer Research.* 70(15) Pp 6368-6376. 2010.

34. Liu S, Wrosch C, Miller G. Pruessner J. **Self-esteem change and diurnal cortisol secretion in older adulthood.** *Psychoneuroendocrinology.* 41; Pp 111-120. 2014.

35. Lovallo W, Al'Absi M, Blick K, Whitsett T, Wilson M. **Stress-like adrenocorticotropin responses to caffeine in young healthy men.** *Pharmacology, Biochemistry, and Behavior.* 55(3); Pp 365-369. 1996.

36. Lovallo W, Whitsett T, al'Absi M, Sung B, Vincent A, Wilson M. **Caffeine stimulation of cortisol secretion across the waking hours in relation to caffeine intake levels.** *Psychosom Med.* 67(5); Pp 734-739. 2005.

37. Malik V, Popkin B, Bray G, Despres J, Hu F. **Sugar sweetened beverages, obesity, type 2 diabetes and cardiovascular disease risk.** *Circulation.* 121(11); Pp 1356-1364. 2010.
38. Maresh C, Whittlesey M, Armstrong L, Yamamoto L, Judelson D, Fish K, Casa D, Kabouras S, Castracane V. **Effect of hydration state on testosterone and cortisol response to training-intensity exercise in collegiate runners.** *International Journal of Sports Medicine.* 27(10); Pp 765-770. 2006.
39. Marinac C, Sears D, Natarajan L, Gallo L, Breen C, Patterson R. **Frequency and circadian timing of eating may influence biomarkers of inflammation and insulin resistance associated with breast cancer risk.** *PLoS One.* 10(8); 2015.
40. Markus R, Panhuysen G, Tuiten A, Koppeschaar H. **Effects of food on cortisol and mood in vulnerable subjects under controllable and uncontrollable stress.** *Physiol Behav.* 70(3-4); Pp 333-342. 2000.
41. Martens M, Rutters F, Lemmens S, Born J, Westerterp-lantenga M. **Effects of single macronutrients on serum cortisol concentrations in normal weight men.** *Physiol Behav.* 101(5); Pp 563-567. 2010.
42. Matyjaszek-Matuszek B, Lenart-Lipinska M, Wozniakowska E. **Clinical implications of vitamin D deficiency.** *Prz Menopauzainy.* 14(2); Pp 75-81. 2015.
43. Mazur A, Booth A. **Testosterone and dominance in men.** *Behavioral and Brain Sciences.* 21; Pp 353-397. 1998.
44. McClain C, Mcclain M, Boosalis M, Hennig B. **Zinc and stress response.** *Scand J Work Environ Health.* 19(1); Pp 132-133. 1993.
45. Nielson F, Johnson L, Zeng H. **Magnesium supplementation improves indicators of low magnesium status and inflammatory stress in adults older than 51 years with poor quality of sleep.** *Magnesium Research.* 23(3); Pp 158-168. 2010.
46. Plazza J, Charles S, Stawski R, Almeida D. **Age and the association between negative affective states and diurnal cortisol.** *Psychology of Aging.* 28(1); Pp 47-56. 2013
47. Prenderville J, Kennedy P, Dinan T, Cryan J. **Adding fuel to the fire: the impact of stress on the ageing brain.** *Trends in Neurosciences.* 38(1); Pp 13-25. 2015.
48. Quraishi S, Camargo C. **Vitamin D in acute stress and critical illness.** *Curr Opin Clin Nutr Metab Care.* 15(6); Pp 625-634. 2012.
49. Rayssiguier R, Libako P, Nowacki W, Rock E. **Magnesium deficiency and metabolic syndrome: Stress and inflammation may reflect calcium activation.** *Magnesium Research.* 23(2); Pp 73-80. 2010.

50. Riskind J, Gotay C. **Physical posture: Could it have regulatory or feedback effects on motivation and emotion.** *Motivation and Emotion.* 6; Pp 273-298. 1982.

51. Rohleder N, Kirschbaum C. **The hypothalamic-pituitary-adrenal (HPA) axis in habitual smokers.** *International Journal of Psychophysiology.* 59(3); Pp 236-243. 2006.

52. Sakaguchi K, Mehta N, Abdallah E, Forgione A, Hirayama H, Kawasaki T, Yokoyama A. **Examination of the relationship between mandibular position and body posture.** *Cranio.* 25(4); Pp 237-249. 2007.

53. Sartori S, Whittle N, Hetzenauer A, Singewald N. **Magnesium deficiency induces anxiety and HPA axis dysregulation: Modulation by therapeutic drug treatment.** *Neuropharmacology.* 62(1); Pp 304-312. 2012.

54. Schug T, Janesick A, Blumberg B, Heindel J. **Endocrine disrupting chemicals and disease susceptibility.** *J Steroid Biochem Mol Biol.* 127(3-5); Pp 204-215. 2011.

55. Shames R, Shames KH. **Thyroid Power.** *Harper Resource.* New York, NY. 2001.

56. Skoluda N, Dettenborn L, et al. **Elevated hair cortisol concentrations in endurance athletes.** *Psychoneuroendocrinology.* September 2011.

57. Sonia C Dumoulin, Bertrand P Perret, Antoine P Bennet and Philippe J Caron. **Opposite effects of thyroid hormones on binding proteins for steroid hormones (sex hormone-binding globulin and corticosteroid-binding globulin) in humans.** *European Journal of Endocrinology.* Vol 132, Issue 5, 594-598, 1995.

58. Sonja Y. Hess, Michael B. Zimmermann, Myrtha Arnold, Wolfgang Langhans and Richard F. Hurrell. **Iron Deficiency Anemia Reduces Thyroid Peroxidase Activity in Rats.** *The Journal of Nutrition.* 132(7); Pp 1951-1955. 2002.

59. *Spreng M.* **Possible health effects of noise induced cortisol increase.** *Noise Health. 2(7); Pp 59-64. 2000.*

60. Stanhope K, Schwarz J, Keim N, et al. **Consuming fructose-sweetened, not glucose-sweetened, beverages, increases visceral adiposity and lipids and decreases insulin sensitivity in overweight/obese humans.** *Journal of Clinical Investigation.* 118(5); Pp 1322-1334. 2009.

61. Stanhope K, Havel P. **Endocrine and metabolic effects of consuming beverages sweetened with fructose, glucose, sucrose, or high fructose corn syrup.** *American Journal of Clinical Nutrition.* 88(6); Pp 1733-1737. 2011.

62. Stanhope K, Bremer A, Medici V, Nakajima K, Ito Y, Nakano T, Chen G, Fong T, Lee V, Menorca R, Keim N, Havel P. **Consumption of fructose and high fructose corn syrup increase postprandial**

triglycerides, LDL-cholesterol, and apolipoprotein-B in young men and women. *The Journal of Clinical Endocrinology and Metabolism.* 96(10); Pp 596-605. 2011

63. Stanhope K. **Sugar consumption, metabolic disease and obesity: the state of the controversy.** *Critical Reviews in Clinical Laboratory Science.* 53(1); Pp 52-67. 2016.

64. Stenius F, Borres M, Bottai M, Lilia G, Lindblad F, Pershagen G, Schevnius A, Swartz J, Theorell T, Alm J. **Salivary cortisol levels and allergy in children: the ALADDIN birth cohort.** *The Journal of Allergy and Clinical Immunology.* 128(6); Pp 1335-1339. 2011.

65. Strack F. **Proprioceptive determinants of emotional and nonemotional feelings.** *Journal of Personality and Social Psychology.* 64; Pp 211-220. 1993.

66. Strack F, Martin L, Stepper S. **Inhibiting and facilitating conditions of the human smile: a nonobtrusive test of facial feedback hypothesis.** *Journal of Personality and Social Psychology.* 54; Pp 768-777. 1998

67. Talbott S. Two food additives to avoid. **The Cortisol Connection Diet.** www.thecortisolconnectiondiet.com

68. Tecco S, Salini V, Tete S, Festa F. **Effects of anterior cruciate ligament injury on muscle activity of head, neck and trunk muscles: a cross sectional evaluation.** *Cranio.* 25(3); Pp 177-185. 2007.

69. Tomiyama A, Mann T, Vinas D, Hunger J, Dejager J, Taylor S. **Low calorie dieting increases cortisol.** *Psychosomatic Medicine.* 72(4); Pp 357-364. 2010.

70. Wang J, Korczykowski M, Rao H, Fan Y, Pluta J, Gur R, McEwen B, Detre J. **Gender difference in neural response to psychological stress.** *Soc Cogn Affect Neurosci.* 2(3); Pp 227-239. 2007.

71. Westerdahl J, Ingvar C, Masback A, Olsson H. **Sunscreen use and malignant melanoma.** *International Journal of Cancer.* 87(1); Pp 145-150. 2000.

72. Wilson J, Adrenal Fatigue Team. **Food allergies, sensitivities and adrenal fatigue.** *www.adrenalfitigue.org.* November 11, 2009.

73. Yang Q, Zhang Z, Gregg E, Flanders W, Merritt R, Hu F. **Added sugar intake and cardiovascular diseases mortality among US adults.** *JAMA International Medicine.* 174(4); Pp 516-524. 2014.

Chapter 2 References

1. Block J, He Y, Zasiavsky A, Ding L, Ayanian J. **Psychosocial stress and change in weight among US adults.** *The American Journal of Epidemiology.* 170(2); Pp 181-192. 2009.
2. Carson S. **Stretching your Stress Out- Meet your Psoas.** www.ekhartyoga.com. March 13, 2014.
3. Cohen S, Deverts D, Doyle W, Miller G, Frank E, Rabin B, Turner R. **Chronic stress, glucocorticoid receptor resistance, inflammation, and disease risk.** *PNAS.* 109(16); Pp 5995-5999. 2012.
4. Drapeau V, Therrien F, Richard D, Tremblay A. **Is visceral obesity a physiological adaptation to stress?** *Panminerva Medica.* 45(3); Pp 189-195. 2003.
5. Ebrecht M, Hextall J, Kirtley L, Taylor A, Dyson M, Weinman J. **Perceived stress and cortisol levels predict speed of wound healing in healthy male adults.**
6. Freedman R, Ianni P. **Role of cold and emotional stress in Raynaud's disease and scleroderma.** *British Medical Journal.* 287(6404); Pp 1499-1502. 1983.
7. Jacka FN et al. **A randomised controlled trial of dietary improvement for adults with major depression (the 'SMILES' trial).** *BMC Medicine* 15(23). 2017.
8. Kamani J. **Hip Flexor Tightness Linked to Chronic Injuries in Student Athlete Runners.** National Scholastic Athletics Foundation. Feb 15, 2015.
9. Larson A, Pardo J, Pasley J. **Review of overlap between thermoregulation and pain modulation in fibromyalgia.** *Clinical Journal of Pain.* 30(6); Pp 544-555. 2014.
10. Moreno-Smith M, Lutgendorf S, Sood A. **Impact of stress on cancer metastasis.** *Future Oncology.* 6(12); Pp 1863-1881. 2010.
11. Shatney L. **How the Adrenals Affect Muscles, Ligaments, and Joints in the Body.** www.Divinehealthfromtheinsideout.com. March 8, 2012.
12. Soffer L, Dorfman R, Gabrilove J. **The human adrenal gland.** Lea and Febiger. Philadelphia, PA. 1961.
13. Thieme G. **Stretching and Strengthening Exercises.** *Thieme Medical Publishers.* New York, NY. 1991.

Chapter 3 References

1. Altman R, Marcussen K. **Effects of a ginger extract on knee pain in patients with osteoarthritis.** *Arthritis Rheum.* 44(11) Pp 2531-2538. 2001.

2. Ammon H. **Boswellic acids in chronic inflammatory disease.** *Planta Med.* 72(12); Pp 1100-1116. 2006.

3. Andrade R, Marino M, Marin D, Camacho G, Caballero M, Marino M. **Variations in urine excretion of steroid hormones after an acute session and after a 4-week programme of strength training.** *European Journal of Applied Physiology.* 99(1); Pp 65-71. 2007.

4. Andrade C, Aswath A, Chaturvedi S, Srinivasa M, Raguram R. **A double-blind, placebo-controlled evaluation of the anxiolytic efficacy ff an ethanolic extract of withania somnifera.** *Indian Journal of Psychiatry.* 42(3); Pp 295-301. 2000.

5. Backhouse S, Biddle S, Williams C. **The influence of water ingestion during prolonged exercise on affect.** *Appetite.* 48(2); Pp 193-198. 2007.

6. Barbadoro P, Anninio I, Ponzio E, Romanelli R, D'Errico M, Prospero E, Minelli A. **Fish oil supplementation reduces cortisol basal levels and perceived stress: a randomized, placebo-controlled trial in abstinent alcoholics.** *Mol Nutr Food Res.* 57(6); Pp 1110-1114. 2013.

7. Beaven C, Gill N, Ingram J, Hopkins W. **Acute salivary hormone responses to complex exercise bouts.** *Journal of Strength and Conditioning Research.* 25(4); Pp 1072-1078. 2011.

8. Berk L, Tan S, Fry W, Napier B, Lee J, Hubbard R, Lewis J, Eby W. **Neuroendocrine and stress hormone changes during mirthful laughter.** *American Journal of Medical Science.* 298(6); Pp 390-396.1989.

9. Brody S, Preut R, Schommer K, Schurmeyer T. **A randomized controlled trial of high dose ascorbic acid for reduction of blood pressure, cortisol, and subjective responses to psychological stress.** *Psychopharmacology.* 159(3); Pp 319-324. 2002.

10. Carney D, Cuddy A, Yap A. **Power Posing: Brief nonverbal displays affect neuroendocrine levels and risk tolerance.** *Psychological Science Online.* Pp 1-6. 2010.

11. Cases J, Ibarra A, Feuillerre N, Roller M, Sukkar S. **Pilot trials of Melissa officinalis L. leaf extract in the treatment of volunteers suffering from mild-to-moderate anxiety disorders and sleep disturbances.** *Mediterranean Journal of Nutrition and Metabolism.* 4(3); Pp 211-218. 2011.

12. Chandrasekhar K, Kapoor J, Anishetty S. **A prospective, randomized double-blind, placebo-controlled study of safety and efficacy of a high-concentration full-spectrum extract of ashwagandha root in reducing stress and anxiety in adults.** *Indian Journal of Psychological Medicine.* 34(3); Pp 255-262. 2012.

13. Childs E, de Wit H. **Regular exercise is associated with emotional resilience to acute stress in healthy adults.** *Frontiers in Physiology.* 5(161); Pp 1-7. 2014.

14. Choi J, Woo T, Yoon S, Compomayor dela P, Choi Y, Ahn H, Lee Y, Yu G, Cheong J. **Red ginseng supplementation more effectively alleviates psychological than physical fatigue.** *Journal of Ginseng Research.* 35(3); Pp 331-338. 2011.

15. Cohen M. **Tulsi – *Ocimum sanctum*: A herb for all reasons.** *Journal of Ayurvedic and Integrative Medicine.* 5(4); Pp 251-259. 2014.

16. Cooley K, Szczurko O, Perri D, Mills E, Bernhardt B, Zhou Q, Seely D. **Naturopathic care for anxiety: a randomized controlled trial ISRCTN78958974.** *PLoS One.* 4(8); e6628. 2009.

17. Cotman C, Berchtold N. **Exercise: a behavioral intervention to enhance brain health and plasticity.** *Trends in Neuroscience.* 25(6); Pp 295-301. 2002.

18. Digdon N, Koble A. **Effects of constructive worry, imagery distraction, and gratitude interventions on sleep quality: a pilot trial.** *Applied Psychology: Health and Well-Being.* 3(2); Pp 193-206. 2011.

19. Dubois O, Salamon R, Germain C, Poirier MF, Vaugeois C, Banwarth B, Mouaffak F, Galinowski A, Olié JP. **Balneotherapy versus paroxetine in the treatment of generalized anxiety disorder.** *Complement Ther Med.* 18(1): Pp 1-7. 2010.

20. Edwards D, Heuffelder A, Zimmerman A. **Therapeutic effects and safety of Rhodiola rosea extract WS ® 1375 in subjects with life-stress symptoms—results of an open-label study.** *Phytotherapy Research.* 26(8); Pp 1220-1225. 2012.

21. Emmons R, McCullough M. **Counting blessings versus burdens: an experimental investigation of gratitude and subjective well-being in daily life.** *Journal of Personality and Social Psychology.* 84(2); Pp 377-389. 2003.

22. Excoffon L, Guillaume Y, Woronoff -Lemsi M, Andre C. **Magneisum effect on testosterone-SHBG association studied by a novel molecular chromatography approach.** *Journal of Pharmaceutical and Biomedical Analysis.* 49(2); Pp 175-180. 2009.

23. Farhanghi M, Mahboob S, Ostadrahimi A. **Obesity induced magnesium deficiency can be treated by vitamin D**

supplementation. *The Journal of the Pakistan Medical Association.* 59(4); Pp 258-261. 2009.

24. Feliu-Hemmelmann K, Monsalve F, Rivera C. **Melissa officinalis and Passiflora caerulea infusion as psychological stress decreaser.** *International Journal of Clinical and Experimental Medicine.* 6(6);Pp 444-451. 2013.

25. Field T, Hernandez-Reif M, Diego M, Schanberg S, Kuhn C. **Cortisol decreases and serotonin and dopamine increase following massage therapy.** *The International Journal of Neuroscience.* 115(10); Pp 1397-1413. 2005.

26. Field T, Field T, Cullen C, Largie S, Diego M, Schanberg S, Kuhn C. **Lavender bath oil reduces stress and crying and enhances sleep in very young infants.** *Early human development.* 84(6); Pp 399-401. 2008.

27. Fraenkel L, Bogardus S, Concato J, Wittink D. **Treatment options in knee osteoarthritis: the patient's perspective.** *Arch Intern Med.* 164(12); Pp 1299-1304. 2004.

28. Fukui H, Toyoshima K, Komaki R. **Psychological and neuroendocrinological effects of odor of saffron (Crocus sativus).** *Phytomedicine.* 18(8-9); Pp 726-730. 2011.

29. Gabel V, Maire M, Reichert C, Chellappa S, Schmidt C,m Hommes V, Viola A, Cajochen C. **Effects of artificial dawn and morning blue light on daytime cognitive performance, well-being, cortisol and melatonin levels.** *Chronobiology International.* 30(8); Pp 988-997. 2013.

30. Garrido M, Espino J, Gonzalez-Gomez D, Lozano M, Barriga C, Paredes S, Rodriguez A. **The consumption of a Jerte Valley cherry product in humans enhances mood, and increases 5-hydroxyindoleacetic acid but reduces cortisol levels in urine.** *Experimental Gerontology.* 47(8); Pp 573-580. 2012

31. Goel N, Kim H, Lao R. **An olfactory stimulus modifies nighttime sleep in young men and women.** *Chronobiology International.* 22(5); Pp 889-904.2005.

32. Gupta I, Gupta V, Parihar A, Gupta S, Ludtke R, Safavhi H, Ammon H. **Effects of Bowellia Serrata gum resin in patients with bronchial asthma: results of a double-blind, placebo-controlled, 6 week clinical study.** *Eur J Med Res.* 3(11); Pp 511-514. 1998.

33. Haskell C, Robertson B, Kennedy D, Milne A, Wetherell M. **Chewing gum alleviates negative mood and reduces cortisol during acute laboratory psychological stress.** *Physiology and Behavior.* 97(3-4); Pp 304-312. 2009.

34. Henkel R, Wang R, Bassett S, Chen T, Liu N, Zhu Y, Tambi M. **Tongkat Ali as a potential herbal supplement for physically active male and female seniors—a pilot study.** *Phytotherapy Research.* 28(4); Pp 544-550. 2014.

35. Isaacs et al. **Exercise and the brain: angiogenesis in the adult rat cerebellum after vigorous physical activity and motor skill learning.** *Journal of Cereb. Blood Flow Metab.* 12; Pp 110-119. 1992.

36. Jesova D, Duncko R, Lassanova M, Kriska M, Moncek F. **Reduction of rise in blood pressure and cortisol release during stress by Ginkgo biloba extract (EGb761) in healthy volunteers.** *Journal of Physiology and Pharmacology.* 53(3); Pp 337-348. 2002.

37. Kawabata K, Kawai Y, Terao J. **Suppressive effect of quercitin on acute stress-induced hypothalamic-pituitary-adrenal axis response in Wistar rats.** *The Journal of Nutritional Biochemistry.* 21(5); Pp 374-380. 2010.

38. Kimura K, Ozeki M, Juneia L, Ohira H. **L-Theanine reduces psychological and physiological stress responses.** *Biological Psychology.* 74(1); Pp 39-45. 2007.

39. Kraft T, Pressman S. **Grin and bear it: the influence of manipulated facial expressions on the stress response.** *Psychol Sci.* 23(11); Pp 1372-1378. 2012.

40. Keller U, Szinnal G, Bilz S, Berneis K. **Effects of changes in hydration on protein, glucose and lipid metabolism in man: impact on health.** *European Journal of Clinical Nutrition.* 57(2); Pp S69-74. 2003.

41. Lau B, Lee J, Li Y, Fung S, Sang Y, Shen J, Chang R, So K. **Polysaccharides from wolfberry prevents corticosterone-induced inhibition of sexual behavior and increases neurogenesis.** *PLoS One.* 7(4); e33374. 2012.

42. Laurin D. **Physical activity and risk of cognitive impairment and dementia in elderly persons.** *Arch. Neurol.* 58; Pp 498-504. 2001.

43. Lee P. **Vitamin D metabolism and deficiency in critical illness.** *Best Pract Res Clin Endocrinol Metab.* 25; Pp 769-781. 2011.

44. Lewith G, Godfrey A, Prescott P. **A single-blinded, randomized pilot study evaluating the aroma of Lavendula augustifolia as a treatment for mild insomnia.** *Journal of Alternative and Complementary Medicine.* 11(4); Pp 631-637. 2005.

45. MacLean C, Walton K, Wenneberg S, Levitsky D, Mandarino J, Waziri R, Hillis S, Schneider R. **Effects of the Transcendental Meditation program on adaptive mechanisms: changes in hormone levels and responses to stress after 4 months of practice.** *Psychoneuroendocrinology.* 22(4); Pp 277-295. 1997.

46. Matsumura K, Yamakoshi T, Noguchi H, Rolfe P, Matsuoka Y. **Fish consumption and cardiovascular response during mental stress.** *BMC Research Notes.* 13(5);Pp 288. 2012.

47. Masteikova R, Bernatoniene J, Bernatoniene R, Valziene S. **Antiradical activities of the extract of passiflora incarnate.** *Acta Pol Pharm.* 65(5); Pp 577-583. 2008.

48. Matyjaszek-Matuszek B, Lenart-Lipinska M, Wozniakowska E. **Clinical implications of vitamin D deficiency.** *Prz Menopauzainy.* 14(2); Pp 75-81. 2015.

49. Mazur A, Booth A. **Testosterone and dominance in men.** *Behavioral and Brain Sciences.* 21; Pp 353-397. 1998.

50. Meinick, M. **How does exercise reduce stress.** *The Huffington Post.* 2013.

51. Nakhostin-Roohi B, Babaei P, Rahmani-Nia F, Bohlooli S. **Effect of vitamin C supplementation on lipid perioxidation, muscle damage and inflammation after 30-min exercise at 75% VO2 max.** *Journal of Sports Medicine and Physical Fitness.* 48(2); Pp 217-224. 2008.

52. Nemeth M, Millesi E, Wagner K, Wallner B. **Effects of diets high in unsaturated fatty acids on socially induced stress responses in guinea pigs.** *PLoS One.* 10(3): e0120188. 2014.

53. Nielson F, Johnson L, Zeng H. **Magnesium supplementation improves indicators of low magnesium status and inflammatory stress in adults older than 51 years with poor quality of sleep.** *Magnesium Research.* 23(3); Pp 158-168. 2010.

54. Oi Y, Imafuku M, Shishido C, Kominato Y, Nishimura S, Iwai K. **Garlic supplementation increases testicular testosterone and decreases plasma corticostereone in rats fed a high protein diet.** *The Journal of Nutrition.* 131(8); Pp 2150-2156. 2001.

55. Oi-Kano Y, Kawada T, Watanabe T, Koyama F, Watanabe K, Senbongi R, Iwai K. **Oleuropein supplementation increases urinary noradrenaline and testicular testosterone levels and decreases plasma corticosterone levels in rats fed high-protein diet.** *Journal of Nutritional Biochemistry.* 24(5); Pp 887-893. 2013.

56. Olsson E, von Scheele B, Panossian A. **A randomized, double blind, placebo controlled, parallel group study of the standardized extract shr-5 of the roots of Rhodiola rosea in the treatment of subjects with stress-related fatigue.** *Planta Med.* 75(2); Pp 105-112. 2009.

57. Pan Y, Zhang W, Xia X, Kong L. **Effects of icariin on hypothalamic-pituitary-adrenal axis action and cytokine levels in stressed Sprague-Dawley rats.** *Biological and Pharmaceutical Bulletin.* 29(12); Pp 2399-2403. 2006.

58. Pawlow L, Jones G. **The impact of abbreviated progressive muscle relaxation on salivary cortisol.** *Biological Psychology.* 60(1); Pp 1-16. 2002.

59. Peters E, Anderson R, Theron A. **Attenuation of increase in circulating cortisol and enhancement of the acute phase protein response in vitamin C supplemented ultramarathoners.** *International Journal of Sports Medicine.* 22(2); Pp 120126. 2001.

60. Quraishi S, Camargo C. **Vitamin D in acute stress and critical illness.** *Curr Opin Clin Nutr Metab Care.* 15(6); Pp 625-634. 2012.

61. Quiroga M, Bongard S, Kreutz G. **Emotional and neurohormonal responses to dancing tango Argentino: The effects of music and partner.** *Music and Medicine.* 1(1); Pp 14-21. 2009.

62. Rayssiguier R, Libako P, Nowacki W, Rock E. **Magnesium deficiency and metabolic syndrome: Stress and inflammation may reflect calcium activation.** *Magnesium Research.* 23(2); Pp 73-80. 2010.

63. Rimmele U, Spillmann M, Bartschi C, Wolf O, Weber C, Ehlert U, Wirtz P. **Melatonin improves memory acquisition under stress independent of stress hormone release.** *Psychopharmacology.* 202(4); Pp 663-672. 2009.

64. Riskind J, Gotay C. **Physical posture: Could it have regulatory or feedback effects on motivation and emotion.** *Motivation and Emotion.* 6; Pp 273-298. 1982.

65. Safarinejad M, Safarinejad S. **Efficacy of selenium and/or N-acetyl-cysteine for improving semen parameters in infertile men: a double-blind, placebo controlled, randomized study.** *Journal of Urology.* 181(2); Pp 741-751. 2009.

66. Sancho R, Lucena C, Macho A, Calzado M, Mlanco-Moline M, Minassi A, Appendino G, Munoz E. **Immunosuppressive activity of capsaicinoids: capsiate derived from sweet peppers inhibits NF-kappaB activation and is a potent anti-inflammatory compound in vivo.** *Eur J Immunol.* 32(6); Pp 1753-1763. 2002.

67. Savorwan W, Siripornpanich V, Piriyapunyaporn T, Hongatanaworakit T, Kotchabhakdi N, Ruangrungsi N. **The effects of lavender oil inhalation on emotional states, autonomic nervous system, and brain electrical activity.** *Journal of the Medical Association of Thailand.* 95(4); Pp 598-606. 2012.

68. Sharp C, Pearson D. **Amino acid supplements and recovery from high-intensity resistance training.** The Journal of Strength and Conditioning Research. 24(4); Pp 1125-1130. 2010.

69. Shevchuk NA. **Adapted cold shower as a potential treatment for depression.** *Med Hypotheses.* 70(5):Pp 995-1001. 2008

70. Smriga M, Ando T, Akutsu M, Furukawa Y, Miwa K, Morinaga Y. **Oral treatment with L-lysine and L-arginine reduces anxiety and basal cortisol levels in healthy humans.** *Biomedical Research.* 28(2); Pp 85-90. 2007

71. Song C, Jung J, Oh J, Kim K. **Effects of Theanine on the release of brain alpha wave in adult males.** *Korean Journal of Nutrition.* 36(9); Pp 918-923. 2003.

72. Spasov A, Wikman G, Mandrikov V, Mironova I, Neumoin V. **A double-blind, placebo-controlled pilot study of the stimulating and adaptogenic effect of Rhodioloa rosea SHR-5 extract on the fatigue of students caused by stress during an examination period with a repeated low-dose regimen.** *Phytomedicine.* 7(2); Pp 85-89. 2000.

73. Starks, Michael, et al. **The effect of phosphatidylserine on endocrine response to moderate intensity exercise.** *Journal of the International Society of Sports Nutrition.* 5(11); 2008.

74. Stepper S, Strack F. **Proprioceptive determinants of emotional and nonemotional feelings.** *Journal of Personality and Social Psychology.* 64; Pp 211-220. 1993.

75. Strack F, Martin L, Stepper S. **Inhibiting and facilitating conditions of the human smile: a nonobtrusive test of facial feedback hypothesis.** *Journal of Personality and Social Psychology.* 54; Pp 768-777. 1998.

76. Talbott S, Talbott J, Pugh M. **Effect of Magnolia offinalis and Phellodendron amurense (Relora ®) on cortisol and psychological mood state in moderately stressed subjects.** *Journal of International Society of Sports Nutrition.* 10(1); Pp 37. 2013.

77. Talbott S, Talbott J, George A, Pugh M. **Effect of Tongkat Ali on stress hormones and psychological mood state in moderately stressed subjects.** *The Journal of International Society of Sports Nutrition.* 10(1); Pp 28. 2013.

78. Toda M, Morimoto K, Nagasawa S, Kitamura K. **Change in salivary physiological stress markers by spa bathing.** *Biomedical Research.* 27: Pp 11–14. 2006.

79. Tokuyama W, et al. **BDNF upregulation during declarative memory formation in monkey inferior temporal cortex.** *Nat Neurosci.* 3;Pp 1134-1142. 2000.

80. Trumble B, Cummings D, O'Connor K, Holman D, Smith E, Kaplan H, Gurven M. **Age-dependent increases in male salivary testosterone during horticultural activity among Tsimane forager-farmers.** *Evolution and Human Behavior.* 34(5); Pp 350-357. 2013.

81. von Kanel R, Meister R, Arpagaus A, Treichler S, Kuebler U, Huber S, Ehlert U. **Dark chocolate intake buffers stress reactivity in humans.**

Journal of the American College of Cardiology. 63(21); Pp 2297-2299. 2014.

82. van Praag H, et al. **Running enhances neurogenesis, learning, and long term presentation in mice.** *Proc Natl Acad Sci USA.* 96; Pp 13427-13431. 1999.

83. Woelk H, Schlafke S. **A multi-center, double-blind, randomized study of the Lavender oil preparation Silexan in comparison to Lorazepam for generalized anxiety disorder.** *Phytomedicine.* 17(2); Pp 94-99. 2010.

84. Yamamoto K, Aso Y, et al. **Autonomic, neuro-immunological and psychological responses to wrapped warm footbaths—a pilot study.** *Complementary Therapies in Clinical Practice.* 14: Pp 195–203. 2008.

85. Young J, Florkowski C, Molyneux S, McEwan R, Frampton C, Nicholls M, Scott R, George P. **A randomized, double-blind, placebo-controlled crossover study of coenzyme Q10 therapy in hypertensive patients with the metabolic syndrome.** *American Journal of Hypertension.* 25(2); Pp 261-270. 2012.

86. Zschucke E, Renneberg B, Dimeo F, Wustenberg T, Strohle A. **The stress buffering effect of acute exercise: evidence for HPA axis negative feedback.** *Psychoneuroendocrinology.* 51. PP 414-425. 2015.

Chapter 4 References

1. Abbasi B1, Kimiagar M, Sadeghniiat K, Shirazi MM, Hedayati M, Rashidkhani B. **The effect of magnesium supplementation on primary insomnia in elderly: A double-blind placebo-controlled clinical trial.** *The Journal of Research in Medical Sciences.* 17(12); Pp 1161-1169. 2012.

2. Andrade R, Marino M, Marin D, Camacho G, Caballero M, Marino M. **Variations in urine excretion of steroid hormones after an acute session and after a 4-week programme of strength training.** *European Journal of Applied Physiology.* 99(1); Pp 65-71. 2007.

3. Digdon N, Koble A. **Effects of constructive worry, imagery distraction, and gratitude interventions on sleep quality: a pilot trial.** *Applied Psychology: Health and Well-Being.* 3(2); Pp 193-206. 2011.

4. Hales B, Pronovost P. **The checklist – a tool for error management and performance improvement.** *Journal of Critical Care.* 21(3); Pp 231-235. 2006.

5. Isaacs et al. **Exercise and the brain: angiogenesis in the adult rat cerebellum after vigorous physical activity and motor skill learning.** *Journal of Cereb. Blood Flow Metab.* 12; Pp 110-119. 1992.

6. Laurin D. **Physical activity and risk of cognitive impairment and dementia in elderly persons.** *Arch. Neurol.* 58; Pp 498-504. 2001.

7. Mudallal Z. **People who make their beds in the morning are happier and are more productive.** *Elite Daily.com. Science Says.* May 7, 2015.

8. Pawlow L, Jones G. **The impact of abbreviated progressive muscle relaxation on salivary cortisol.** *Biological Psychology.* 60(1); Pp 1-16. 2002.

9. Saxbe D, Repetti R. **No Place Like Home: Home Tours Correlate With Daily Patterns of Mood and Cortisol.** *Personality and Social Psychology Bulletin.* 36 (1); Pp 71-81. 2010.

10. Shevchuk NA. **Adapted cold shower as a potential treatment for depression.** *Med Hypotheses.* 70(5):Pp 995-1001. 2008

11. Tokuyama W, et al. **BDNF upregulation during declarative memory formation in monkey inferior temporal cortex.** *Nat Neurosci.* 3;Pp 1134-1142. 2000.

12. van Praag H, et al. **Running enhances neurogenesis, learning, and long term presentation in mice.** *Proc Natl Acad Sci USA.* 96; Pp 13427-13431. 1999.

www.ingramcontent.com/pod-product-compliance
Lightning Source LLC
Chambersburg PA
CBHW021340290326
41933CB00037B/310